All EMF*d Up

(*ElectroMagneticField)

My Journey through Wireless Radiation Poisoning

Plus

How you can Protect Yourself

by Anne Mills

with notes by Eric Mills & Lloyd Morgan

*All EMF*d Up*

(*Electromagnetic Fields)
My Journey through Wireless Radiation Poisoning
  Plus - How You Can Protect Yourself

***Copyright**[1]* **© *2019 Anne Mills* -**All rights reserved.
No part of this book may be reproduced in any form or by any electronic or mechanical means, including information storage and retrieval systems, without permission in writing from the publisher, except by reviewers, who may quote brief passages in a review.
RedwoodPortal@Yahoo.com

For Permission to use material from other works:
Photos by Eric Mills
Cover design and images by Akeson Design

Printed in the United States of America
Published by Redwood Portal Publishing

Although the author and publisher have made every effort to ensure that the information in this book was correct at press time, the author and publisher do not assume and hereby disclaim any liability to any party for any loss, damage, or disruption caused by errors or omissions, whether such errors or omissions result from negligence, accident, or any other cause.

ISBN 978-1-7339507-0-1

1. Environmentally induced diseases – Alternative treatment.
2. Environmental illness. 3. Electromagnetic Sensitivity. 4. Microwave Sickness. 5. Technology – health and safety. 6. Electro-pollution. 7. Environmental pollution.
8. Cell phones and cancer risks. 9. Memoirs

Important Information

Part 1 Disclaimer: This book is a true story, with real life events. There were some in this true story whose lives or livelihoods' were threatened by 'powers that be', so some names and locations have been changed in an effort to protect them and their families. I may have changed some identifying characteristics and details such as physical properties, occupations and places of residence. I would like to thank my friends and family portrayed in this book for letting me share this story. This book is not intended to hurt anyone, and I regret any unintentional harm resulting from publishing and marketing All EMF*d Up.

Part 2 Disclaimer: The contents of this book are based on perspectives gained from my experiences. I have tried to notate ownership of individual research papers. The sharing of my experiences is not meant as medical advice nor a tool for self-diagnosis. This book is not intended as a substitute for the medical advice of physicians. Please come to decisions for your health based on your own research and in partnership with your physician. If you are pregnant, taking medications or have any pre-existing conditions, please consult with your health care professional prior to experimenting with any personal trials I might have shared. Please do not put off seeing a physician if you believe you are ill. Thank you. •

Note: This book does not lead to selling online courses or EMF gadgets. I do not work for, consult, own shares in or receive funding from any company or organization that would benefit from this book.

Table of Contents

Introduction   5

Dedication   7

Prologue   9

Part 1

My Journey Through Wireless Radiation Poisoning   11

Part 2

What is ElectroMagnetic Hyper Sensitivity (EHS)   103
    Symptoms   107

How to Protect Your Home and Work Environment   116
    Awareness, Acknowledgement, Avoidance of EMF   116
    Decision, Determination and Cooperation   117
    Using Technology Safely   118
    Protecting your Home from Outside EMF Sources   121
    Protection from Smart Meter   122
    Building Biologist   123
    Why a Radiation Meter is Important   123
    Less Radiation at Work   125

Cell Phones and How to Reduce Radiation   128
    A Little Information on Cell Phone Health Risk   131

EMF Meters and ELF Meters   133
    Radiation Meters   133
    Dirty Electricity and ELF Meters   138

TriField EMF Meter   140

Situational Awareness   142

Living by the Meter   142

Protective Shelters — **147**
- Faraday Shelters — 147
- Fabric Shelter — 149
- Final Faraday Design — 150
- RF Shielding Foil Faraday — 155
- Rolling Faraday Shelter — 158
- EMF Blocking Sleeping Bag — 159

Personal EMF Protection — **161**
- Protective clothing — 162

Traveling Safely with EHS — **170**
- Window Tinting — 171

Healing and Recovery from an EMF poisoning — **174**
- EMF Detox — 179
- EMFs in Pregnancy and with Young Children — 181

Diagnosis, Disability and ADA — **184**
- Diagnosis — 184
- Social Security Disability Insurance – SSDI — 187
- Americans with Disability Act – ADA — 189

Fight or Flight — **194**

Depression — **197**

Eric's Perspective — **205**

Intervention for EHS Access — **211**

The New Normal — **217**

Killing us Softly – — **227**

5G, Cell towers, Smart meters, WiFi in schools — **227**
- Schools: Computers, Yes; Wifi, No ! — 228
- Cell Towers — 229
- "Smart" Utility Meters — 231

Commercial Awareness	234
Against 5G	235
White Zones	**239**
Take-Aways	**242**
Conclusion	**244**
Epilogue	**245**
More Info	**246**

Introduction

Do you suffer from relentless insomnia, tinnitus or sporadic insane headaches? Do you experience puzzling heart palpitations, vertigo or unusual moodiness and depression? Is your physician having a difficult time diagnosing the health issues you've encountered? Your symptoms could be brought on by wireless radiation environmental pollution.

This book is for those that are questioning the safety of wireless radiation and 5G, and interested in knowing how to protect yourself and loved ones. This book is for those who are curious about, think they might have, or are supporting someone who has Electromagnetic Hypersensitivity (EHS), also known as Wireless Radiation Sickness.

The first section of this book is my memoir of how I was poisoned and became ill from man-made electromagnetic frequency radiation (EMF) while living in Europe. I was diagnosed by German physicians in 2006, and guided to recovery. To discover where these radiation emissions were coming from I had to interact with German scientists, physicians and government officials. My next quest was how can I protect myself from these radiation emissions? How can I recover from their substantial ill effects? Why is the government involved, and why have there been threats to researchers and smoke screen letters? This poisoning event left me extremely sensitive to, and unable to live around, anything wireless.

How does one sensitive to EMF live in a world filled with wireless radiation? The second part of this book offers the healing knowledge my physicians from Europe imparted and how our family worked through the issues, dealt with unknowing U.S. physicians and lawyers, unbelieving acquaintances, concerned family and friends. We show how we were able to protect ourselves in our homes, autos, and travel. This book shows how to build a faraday cage and our experience on buying radiation meters. I have a chapter on situational awareness and how to deal with a society blinded by the wireless industry spin. The suggestions in this book are offered as an easy read in how to help yourself, how to protect yourself, how to clean up your immediate surroundings, how to apply for Social Security Disability based on EHS and where you can find more information and scientific studies on the subject.

By sharing this experience, I hope that those that know me will better understand why I worry about them and their future health; that those who are, or think they might be affected by EMF radiation, have a better idea of how to protect themselves and their loved ones; and that those who were curious now have a better understanding and a new compassion for those of us that do suffer from EHS.

As I was poisoned by electromagnetic frequency (EMF) radiation, this is what this book is based on.

I am a survivor. We are the evidence. Please join me in this healing journey.

Note: As there were some in this true story whose lives or livelihoods' were threatened by 'powers that be', some names and locations have been changed, in an effort to protect them.

Dedication

In deepest gratitude and devotion, I would like to dedicate this book to my talented, loving, and supportive husband of over forty years, Eric. While I was so deep in the process of writing, he was always willing to manage the chores, offer moral support and great hugs, and make me take breaks to eat. Thank you to my protector and champion.

Acknowledgements

First I would like to express thanks to all those who upon hearing our story on EMF poisoning, told us "you've got to write this down!", "you've got to write a book", "people have got to know this". If not for their appeals, I would not have thought anyone would have been interested. So, Thank You Lloyd Morgan and all.

My heartfelt thanks to my writing instructor and editor of the first half of this book, Ida Egli, who was kind enough to offer her expertise to polish and improve the quality of my writing. Ida, an author in her own right, gave me much support and encouragement and for that I am grateful. It feels as though it is as important for her, as it is for me, to see this to fruition. Ida is my standard.

I am most thankful to my wonderful friends who pre edited and all those who gave me moral support and suggestions. It was like having my own cheering section. So special thanks to Helen, Judith, Carol, Jennifer, Beth and Phyllis.

Affectionate thanks to my talented brother Eric, for his understanding and protection of my health issues, and sharing of his knowledge of writing. Thank you for the many creative hours you put towards this project.

This is the perfect time to express gratitude to all those in the fast growing contingent of supporters for those of us with ElectroMagnetic Sensitivity or Microwave Sickness. For their tireless pioneering efforts, commitment and drive to bringing more awareness to the negative impacts of Electromagnetic Fields, all things EMF*d Up, Thank You Sandi Maurer, Patricia Burke, Arthur Firstenberg, Eric Windheim, Dr. S.Eberle, Dr. Toril Jelter, Lloyd Morgan, Dr. Martin Pall and all. You are appreciated.

Prologue
Slow Awakening

It is night. I am lying in a fetal position and my eyes are closed, my fists clenched. My body shakes with tremors, like I am cold—but I am not. Or, like my blood is boiling. I can find no comfortable position to help endure the pain. My body aches all over: my hips, my shoulders, my back—as if I've been beaten. And, I'm drenched in sweat.

I recall now that I was on the floor with a blanket and my pillow in the small bathroom in the basement cellar. In this room the humming that is driving me crazy is the quietest. I don't know the time, but because the pain has subsided some, I surmise that the horrific night is over. I am exhausted. My memory flits over the night hours and I find it hard to believe what is there: nausea, headaches that last for only seconds but feel like spikes from an ice pick, loud humming, nose bleeds, and shaking. I feel as though I've ingested ten cups of coffee. My fists are still clenched and when I try to open them it is difficult.

I grab my pillow and blanket and groggily head up the stairs to the bedroom. Then I notice my hands are wet, sticky with blood. My palms are cut with half-moons from my fingernails when I clenched in pain. Again. How many nights will this happen? How long will this madness go on? What is this invisible monster? Where does it come from and where does it go during the day?

I quietly crawl back into the bed I share with my husband, Eric, and try to hold still. He has to work today and needs his sleep. But he notices I've returned to bed. He rolls over " Oh honey, another bad night?" Eric holds me, rocks me, and I inhale the comfort. He whispers "While I am at work, go into town, to that meeting, and see if you can talk to someone who might believe or understand what you are going through." There is nothing he can do to make the bad nights better and I know he feels guilty. I am just so glad the daylight has arrived because the normalcy of the day helps me endure the madness of the night.

Part 1

My Journey Through Wireless Radiation Poisoning

My name is Anne. My husband, Eric, our two cats, and I moved to Bavaria, Germany in 2006. Eric's employer of twenty-eight years, Siemens, is a large electronics firm, and Eric's division makes medical devices for cancer treatments. Eric, as a manager, is tasked with helping move the business from the Bay Area of California to Germany. Our contract is for four years. We are an active, healthy couple, married twenty-seven years. We enjoy travel, motorcycling, hiking and bicycling. This should be a perfect move for us. Our only child, Ian, nineteen-years-old, is attending college in California.

Eric has been assigned to the facility in Erlangen, in the northern part of Bavaria. The home we are renting in Dormitz, a small farming hamlet of about 700 residents, is a short fifteen-minute commute from Erlangen. Having just flown in, we are excited and tired, as we drive in our packed rental car through this small town with cobblestone streets. We pass buildings hundreds of years old but still inhabited. They seem to guard the streets with their block stature and thick stone walls. There are old farmhouses and barns in the middle of town, and it looks like the most common vehicle is the family tractor. We find ourselves following directions up a narrow street to a beautiful white house on the top of a hill.

The house is a newly built four-story (including basement), white with red tile roof, and looks like a castle. When we enter our new home, it feels cavernous compared to our small ranch house back in the Bay Area. Our furniture has not yet arrived, and neither have the two vehicles we had shipped. The massive house, much too big for two people, echoes with our steps. In our amazement we find that the landlord has left a mattress and a dining table with a bench. In the kitchen, on the counter, they have gifted us a small basket containing sausage, crackers and cheese, and a couple candles. Their note reads, "in case the electricity goes out." They leave a phone number. We are so appreciative. We feel welcomed.

Eric began working the following day, and I filled those first days unpacking what little we did bring, practicing my *Deutsch*, and taking walks in the neighborhood to get familiar with our surroundings. The people were friendly. A couple of days later we heard a knock on the door. Opening it we faced seven elderly neighbors and one of their daughters, as translator. They came over to welcome us to the neighborhood. They all wore big smiles, and the women offered us a gift basket containing a round loaf of dark brown bread wrapped in a new kitchen towel, a jar of salt, and a bouquet of fresh garden flowers. As translated, the bread conveyed the wish we never run out of food, the salt so we always had employment and money. What could we say? I was so touched I cried. Smiling I said *"Danke."*

We lived out of suitcases the next month and a half. I felt glad I had thought to bring plates, cups, utensils and towels. We were lacking many household items we hadn't brought or that hadn't yet arrived, so we started going to the weekend *Trodel*, or flea markets. Not only were we able to purchase things we needed immediately for less money than new, but also it was interesting. Many of the items sold at Trodel markets appeared to be antiques, and that lent us the experience of living in a kind of "poor man's museum". Fun. Then, when our household boxes did arrive, it felt like Christmas, opening boxes and unwrapping, once again holding our familiar, useful belongings.

Though we have left friends, family, aging parents, and a home of twenty years in the Bay Area of California, we are looking forward to immersing ourselves in the German culture and traveling every weekend. With the close proximity of neighboring countries, France, Italy, Austria, Hungary, we are close enough to visit them on long weekends. Also, working in Germany, Eric receives six weeks paid vacation and a thirty-five hour workweek. We are eager to take advantage of the ease of travel living in Europe. Customs isn't releasing our cars, so to compensate we purchase an old used Opel, to carry us until our vehicles are released.

    I had left an administrative assistant position and a part-time teaching job at a local wildlife museum to come to Germany. I saw our move and its challenges of everyday life as interesting and fun. I was determined to maintain an open heart and a mind full of wonder. I think I saw this as a chance for personal growth, and I wanted to support Eric in his professional challenge.

    I met an elderly neighbor on the path by our home, Herr Singer. He spoke English due to being held captive in an Allied POW camp during the war. His property abutted ours, and he said I could use an area near our driveway to grow vegetables. In exchange, I re-roofed Herr Singer's little garden house. I tore off the old shingles and his nephew, Jair, our other next-door neighbor, purchased new ones. I looked up on the computer how to replace a roof, and after cleaning the roof with a wire brush, nailed on the new shingles. The roof looked great, and in the deal I now had a little garden area. I had gardened my whole life and didn't want to stop. Herr Singer gave me that opportunity, and I felt great.

    Customs finally delivered our cars. We had shipped them from California in April and now it was August; it was good to see them again. Eric and I had been sport motorcyclists for more than forty years and loved the thrill of a good curvy mountain road. As we did not ship over a motorcycle, Eric purchased a used Cagiva Gran Canyon motorcycle. In August, we toured the Italian Alps for five days on that motorcycle, our first of many such vacations.

Changes to our health September-October, 2006.

I have always known good health. So when faced with alarming symptoms, I felt afraid and confused. We were living in Germany because Eric had a professional contract there. I was slowly learning German so, of course, my language gap left me unable to share easily with those around me. The friends and acquaintances I communicated with back in California were as stumped as I was. Why was I so ill, and why mostly at night? Why wasn't Eric more ill? I had been healthy in June when we arrived from California. What had happened in the last five months? Did I have a genetic disease or one from an environmental influence, like water, mold, or unfamiliar food? Had I suddenly developed a chemical sensitivity?

There were so many questions about the magnified night symptoms, and why during the day I was able to cope as though nothing untoward was happening. I was still able to perform my myriad of chores even though my energy level, strength, and stamina were now taxed. I wanted to present to Eric after his stressful day a welcoming front at home. I did not want him to worry about our finances, bills, laundry, household chores, recycling. Rather, I wanted him to come home to a well-prepared dinner on the table. I had to pull from within myself a determination I had no idea I possessed, to meet the demands of a supportive wife. Eric sometimes worked ten-plus hour days so I was often alone. When we had a working computer I was able to do online searches to try and put a name to my strange physical problems, but I found no viable answers. I had a real mystery going on and I did not like it.

It had started as a humming and whining, of different pitches, at night. I could not locate where these innocuous sounds were coming from, but I conjectured they were emanating from some kind of energy source, perhaps electrical in nature. I walked around in my pajamas from room to room, putting my ear to every working appliance, trying to find the instigator: the refrigerator, the computer, the phones, the freezer, and the oil heating system. Nothing matched the frequency of the hum I was experiencing. The high- pitched whining usually began after I had gone to bed, waking me up at exactly 11:00 PM. The whining did not wake or disturb Eric. I could hear undulations, as the whines got worse towards the half hour, gradually growing quieter closer to the hour. I'd fade to sleep only to be awakened, again at the top of the hour. I began keeping a diary of the humming, naming the sound pitches, and the hum time and their duration. Perhaps if I had been musically trained I would have labeled the hums as *high C* or *D flat*, but I did not have that expertise so I came up with my own labels: *my father's razor*, *water through pipes*, or the low pitch of *garage door opening*.

    At the same time—not making the connection they might be related—I began experiencing heart palpitations, nose bleeds and severe allergy symptoms. My menses abruptly stopped. Both Eric and I started losing hair. Sometimes I was unable to focus and express myself. Me, at a loss for words! I was becoming quite alarmed as I noted all these symptoms in the diary. Eric suffered bouts of upset stomach and nosebleeds. As the humming noise intensified, so did our symptoms. Every night the hums would come on at the top of the hour, and seemingly slowly ramp up in strength, until they felt to be on *high power* at the half-hour, tapering down until almost indiscernible at the three-quarter hour, then on again at the top of the hour. It felt like the noises were giving me a fifteen-minute sleep break.

    The ramping up, coupled with the humming, led me to believe this was definitely an energy-flow problem of some sort. I couldn't see or smell anything out of the ordinary. It happened mainly at night, starting around 10:00 PM. I had no idea what all this meant, and when I mentioned what was happening to my friend Kerstin, also from California, now living in the next hamlet over, she had never heard of anyone having symptoms like mine. Her husband, Uwe, had worked with Eric at Siemens in California. Kerstin suggested I visit the local physician.

I began experiencing pain throughout my body, from my shoulders to my ankles, and in every joint in my hands. Eric was experiencing ill health, as well, but his symptoms were different and not as intense. I supposed this was because he worked ten hours a day—in a different environment. When the noises would wake me, I'd hold still and remain quiet so Eric could continue to sleep, knowing he had to work the next day. Invariably, though, after about fifteen minutes he would wake, complaining of an upset stomach. So in this way I came to realize that even though I was the only one hearing the noises, the *energy*, or whatever it was, the menace was also negatively impacting him.

I still had no idea what these symptoms meant, and I also still felt relatively well during the day, doing my best to ignore my symptoms. But, too, the louder the humming, the sicker I felt. I started keeping a flashlight, notebook, and pen beside the bed to note in my diary the times and durations of the humming and my corresponding symptoms. I thought that if I could nail down the patterns maybe I could deduce what was happening to us. I continued to name the humming sounds, adding a grading system that analyzed the relative intensity of the energy surges numerically, 1 through 10. That might sound overdone, and sometimes it felt that way to me, but I was awake anyway. And this record keeping helped me feel a modicum of control over my weird situation.

By November the humming noise woke me every night at 11:00 PM and lasted six to eight hours solid. I was clearly hearing and feeling an *energy*, an intense buzzing. I was experiencing terrible night sweats now, waking up drenched, my nightshirt, my long hair, the bedding, all wet. I would get up, dry off, change to a new nightshirt and cover the wet of the bed with a towel so I could go back to sleep. When the energy was high I also shook all over with tremors, as though I'd had ten cups of coffee. I was literally vibrating. This was terrible, really scary. After a month of the 11:00 PM, start time it switched to beginning at 2:00 AM, then later, for several weeks, to 1:00 AM, then back to 2:00 AM. The constant was that the humming always lasted six to eight hours.

Then, suddenly, it seemed that the frequency of the hum changed. I became aware of nights when it was clearly worse than other nights and nights when I felt sure there was a greater strength in the hummed frequencies. Somewhere toward the end of November an additional hum was initiated. Where I had previously heard only a deep, low hum, now there was also a higher octave hum similar to *water thru a pipe*. The different noises continued to begin and end at their usual times, but they were distinctly different sounds. This drove me nuts. Should I attribute the strange symptoms these noises caused to menopause and/or insomnia—or credit the *energy* with causation? I might be able to attribute the rapid heartbeats, headaches, and nosebleeds to dry air and stress, but more symptoms were piling up: joint pain, hair loss, pain in my ovaries and breasts. Overall, before, I had felt in good health for a fifty-year-old. No one ever took me for being over thirty-five! Now, suddenly, I felt seventy. What gives?

In December we took the train to Rome for five days. The trip was fun, and unlike at home, I felt fine and I slept well. I was like a new person. Yes! This went some way to convincing me that the health issues we were experiencing were caused by something in our home environment. I realized, too, that I had to start looking outside of the house for an explanation.

We made a decision to move. Eric had been transferred to a different Siemens facility in Kemnath, an hour and a half drive from the house. The vehicles we had shipped over from the states were vintage, and Germany's winter roads were all icy. They salt the roads for traction, and not wanting to subject our old cars to the slushy salt meant Eric drove the newer Opel. So, our vintage autos stayed garaged in the winter, and it seemed so far like it was always winter here. We had brought our own cars and now were unable to use them! We decided to start looking for a house to rent that was closer to Eric's work location.

2007 – Happy New Year

In mid-January, our next-door- neighbor, Jair, ran over to tell us a huge storm was coming the next morning and to make sure things were secured. We then got an email from Kerstin saying the same, "batten down the hatches". Eric and I ran around the yard and pulled inside anything that might blow away or become a missile. Then we went around the interior of the house and lowered all the metal window coverings. We felt glad there were people watching out for us as without television or radio we had no way to get weather reports. I was never good at storms in California, and I wasn't looking forward to this one in Germany. When it hit, the storm was loud and shook the house and foundation. From peeks outside we saw the sky was deep plum-purple and dark as night. Even the huge gutters, the size of five gallon buckets split lengthwise, were not able to hold the deluge of water noisily pouring over their sides. In only a few minutes our patio was under an inch of water. All storms last too long for me, but this one went on into the morning. Every storm I had experienced in California now seemed like a baby tantrum compared to the German barrage of donner and blitz. I immediately learned to love metal shutters.

Diary - Jan 16, 2007. I went into Erlangen (by bus) yesterday. It was beautiful weather and I walked around Erlangen for hours, had lunch, enjoyed the bookstore and strolled through art stores. I even needed sunglasses and had to remove coat, hat, and scarf during my walk. Sweater weather, in January, who'd a thought! Last week, however, the wind blew so hard one of the cherry trees behind our house broke, was twisted off in the middle, probably an eight to ten inch tree! The wind blows so hard up on this ridge that it sounds and shakes like a train idling alongside the house.

Dear Diary – Jan. 18, 2007 What is happening?
I was in the Opel wagon with Eric. I was not sure where we were going or why and I was unable to sit up on my own. I would constantly fall asleep. That is all I remember, and I now wonder how many days were like this. I sleep all day. I don't feel like eating. It's like my body is shutting down. Normally an avid, even addictive, reader, I can't concentrate enough to make sense of what I am reading. I now have no desire to pick up a book as I am not only extremely tired all the time, but nauseated and lightheaded as well. I find myself increasingly frustrated when I can't find words in my head to match my feelings. I forget my train of thought; why did I go into the kitchen? Exhaustion has led me to feel like my main job is horizontally weighing down the couch to keep it from floating away.
I can't make tea anymore!
I walked down the stairs in my sweat pants and shirt from bedroom to kitchen with my ankles and knees very achy. Eric had already gone to work. I remembered the energy— if that is what this is—the previous night had been a high eight out of ten on my mental meter. In the light of day it was easier to pretend everything had been normal. This morning I now felt like I'd run a marathon. The day was cold, as usual, and I felt I needed a cup of nice hot tea, but had no idea how to make tea. Me, a super organized multitasker! I had no idea how to make a cup of tea. What was wrong with me? I stood at the counter trying to concentrate. Okay, Okay. A teapot. Okay. Water. Put water in the teapot. Stunned, losing even my fine grasp of next steps…the stove. A tea bag. I found that I had to say the words out loud because my thoughts were not registering into any action. Not that there is anything wrong with talking with oneself, but I

never had, and this was now an unconscious happening. Where once tea was a simple non-chore, suddenly it was a major work. What was wrong with me? In my frustration and fear, I just sat and cried.

It dawns on me then that I am very ill. My imagination running wild, all kinds of possible scary illnesses race through my mind. I go to the computer and WebMD, and put in my symptoms: insomnia, heart palpitations, night sweats, cessation of menses, headache, skin rash, body aches, vertigo, hair loss, tinnitus, nausea, fatigue, confusion. I get a choice of about twelve different diagnoses, everything from the flu to Parkinson to a drug overdose. I have always been healthy and conscious of the need for a healthy diet and for exercise. I was healthy six months earlier in California. After our vacation to Italy I felt much better. I must be ill due to our environment. But so much has changed since I left home. Weather, totally different from California's sunny days, and the food is not our normal food. Water is different. Air seems fresh. Our neighbors seem fine, and do not speak of ill health issues.

I climb to the third story of the house, up through the attic ladder and door, and look out. The view from the little hill we are perched on is amazing. To the east is a wonderful view of several small colorful hamlets, nestled into a large bowl. The red roofs amid the tree greenery remind me of a bowl of cherries. To the west is a neighbor's house, and next to it an orchard. To the south, beside our back yard, is a dirt road traveled by local farmers on tractors. On the other side of the dirt road lay a small wheat field and a barn, and attached to the small barn, several ugly cell tower masts. Could the cell towers be a factor in our ill health?

Diary- Mid Jan. 2007
One night...
The humming. It is 1:00 AM and the energy intensity is starting to worsen. This has got to stop. Where is it coming from? Who is doing this? Eric is asleep, so I tell him I am going to find out what is making me ill before I am too ill to get dressed. I don't know if he wakes enough to hear or understand. I pull on sneakers and throw on a robe over my PJs, grab my car keys and head out the front door. It is winter, and there is ice on the ground. This is Germany. The Opel wagon, luckily, is easy to start. I creep down the little alley street we are on, and turn right, heading towards where I think the cell antenna that I can see from the house, is located. I presume that as I drive closer to the antenna the humming will get louder, but I don't hear any humming. I drive down the dirt street with the farmhouse on the left and a wheat field on the right. There is our house, on the other side of the wheat field. I turn the car around. What now? I just sit in the dark, in the cold, in front of the barn, and know I'm fighting windmills. I lay my head on the steering wheel and cry. I'm feeling ill and know I must get home. But home offers no answers either.

Another night -
The humming comes on at 11:00 PM and ramps higher and higher, bringing on aches and nausea and headaches. No sleep. I'm wracked in pain. It seems to peak at 11:30 and tapers down to nothing at 11:45. It is off now. I know I will have a fifteen-minute respite until it comes on again at midnight. This will happen again at 1:00 AM, 2:00 AM, 3:00 AM, 4:00 AM and lastly at 5:00 AM. Why is this so predictably timed? Who is needing this energy in the middle of the night? I get up and go to the computer and start doing searches of how cell towers are used. I come across a site that shows how Internet companies offer businesses a way to upload their business documents and

files into the "cloud". This upload takes place when there is not as much demand on the towers...like in the middle of the night. My search takes me to Alice. This is a company that offers businesses upload capability in our area, and amazingly, I am able to see when they are uploading which company. It coincides with my diary notes of times when I am ill, have my symptoms. I print out pages of the times bandwidth is used and by whom. I have no idea how I will use this information, but it vilifies the humming source and validates the timing of my pain.

Another night -
I am so ill. I need to find a place to sleep. I am so, so tired. I grab my pillow and a blanket and start to wander around the three-story house, looking for a place where the humming is not so loud. The bathtub. I lay in the bathtub. It seems to help a little.

Another night -
I want to sleep so badly. I try the bathtub, but tonight the energy is too high. It is winter, but I put on my slippers and go outside and into the garage and I make a bed for myself in our old 1958 MG Magnette. It has a nice big backseat. This seems to help some. I lie there and cry myself to sleep, waking before daybreak to walk back into the house.

Another night -
It is snowing outside, and the energy is very high. I wander into the basement, trying different spaces to find somewhere that has less humming, less pain, but is maybe warmer than the back seat of a car. I try behind the footwell of the winding staircase. I try the little bathroom that is in the basement, in an interior hallway with rooms on either side. Maybe. It is so small I must pull in my feet before I shut the door. No window, but I'm not claustrophobic, I am tired. But the night is not a good one. I am glad there is a toilet so close.

Many nights I just wander around the house, trying to find solace. Many nights I am too ill to sleep. Many nights the insomnia is all encompassing, like the pain, nausea, and tremors. There is no one to help me, and no one to explain what is happening. There is no one to say it will go away or that I will live through this and no one to commiserate and tell me I am not alone. Except Eric. I am so lucky to have Eric and his support. He believes me.

Could the grids I see be a new symptom? I did not know what they were when I first saw them. I was feeling quite ill, like I had a terrible, never-ending flu. But each morning that followed a night of quite heavy energy, I saw before me a grid, or a honeycomb pattern. I would see the grid pattern prior to opening my eyes and focusing. This would last for several minutes, even after I had opened my eyes. I would see a full page, up close, of the grid pattern, as if I was holding graph paper to my face. At first they were just black and white squares in a tight pattern. I had no idea what caused them or why I saw them. Soon enough the simple grid pattern changed. Changes came fast, every week or so, and then the changes slowed. The grids became rectangular, then oblong, then like pointed ovals. Eventually they began to have a dot in the center. Next, I noticed they were no longer black and white, but were, instead, blue or red. After a while the *grids* became connected and elliptical. All this happened only after heavy energy nights. I noted all of this in my diary.

Diary: A lot of learning in a short amount of time. I guess all it takes is one communication with the right person to put one on the right track.

It was the end of January, and I had continued to feel unwell. I still could not figure out the cause. The leaves had fallen from the large oaks in the backyard, opening up a view to the cell tower masts across the field. I went to our next-door neighbor, Jair, who spoke English, and voiced my concerns. I asked him about the cell towers, wondering if they could adversely affect me. I confessed that at night I heard a loud, low hum and because of that I was unable to sleep, my ears ringing all day (tinnitus). "I don't know how much of what I am feeling is associated with these cell towers, Jair, but I need to know if there is a health risk living close to these towers." Jair and I walked over and looked across the field to the barn decorated with cell towers. We also noted that to one side of the wheat field, behind a neighbor's house, was a small antenna. It looked like a tall metal stick, not as foreboding as the towers on the barn. Jair and I wondered together if these could pose a health risk. He said he would look into it.

  Later that day, Jair emailed me a website about amateur radio, or ham radio operation, which is what the smaller antenna was for. He also emailed me a link explaining "electrosmog", plus a site for the Federal Office for Radiation Protection. With the information Jair gave me, I started investigating. I searched online to find out if there were known health dangers associated with cell towers. I would pull up the information in Deutsche, copy the paragraph and paste it into a translation site for German to English. I learned that the cell towers are called "masts" in Germany. I also learned that the masts give off electrosmog or radiation. I found only a few sites and no real support or chat lines. There are no sites defining medical risks from close by masts. I found these sites mainly focused on microwaves:
  www.nomasts.org.uk , www.mastsanity.org.uk , www.powerwatch.org, www.towersanity.org, www.mindfully.org, (none of which are valid sites anymore.)

  From these websites I learned that "electrosmog" radiation energy is dangerous to one's health. The websites mentioned cell towers as health dangers and listed many of my symptoms. I learned that governments encourage the use of cell tower masts. I learned that there is a ton of money invested by the wireless industry connected to the towers. This did not help me understand how to help myself, though, or how to feel better. The knowledge did nothing to mitigate the unimaginable illness that each night brought me.

On the first day of February I rode my bike down to the local "Rathaus" where the mayor and city officials are housed. The mayor, Bernhard Weber, was polite and most helpful, and he spoke English. He looked up phone numbers and contacted a federal agency while I waited, informing me that there were "…three antenna in our close vicinity, one antenna owned by T-Com, one by an "M----" company (I was told not to use their name), and a third antenna on the barn across the field from me owned by someone the federal agency refused to name. The federal agency told us "the masts were all working within legal limits." Certainly in my mind I assumed the federal agency would not allow the masts to operate under conditions that would be harmful to one's health. I still wondered if the night use of these masts was causing my ill health, but I could not be certain. I had no other ideas. Where else could I turn?

Next I rode my bike to see the doctor in our small village. Physicians in Europe see people on short notice. Luckily, Dr. Quentin seemed very competent and nice, spoke a halting English, and said she had no idea what the cause of my various symptoms were. The doctor suggested that, even though I had none of these symptoms a few months ago in California, it was possible I could now be experiencing menopause, arthritis, and stress. When I informed her of the masts about 200 yards away from our house, just across a small wheat field, she got real quiet. After a few moments of thought, she suggested I go to a meeting of citizens against cell tower masts that, amazingly, was going to be held on March 7th, in our town. She believed that someone there would be able to help answer my questions. I had no idea if there would be anyone at the meeting who spoke English, but I was not going to let this opportune meeting pass me by. Though March seemed a long time to wait for answers, I had no choice. Dr. Quentin said she would see me there.

> Feb.4, 2007- email:
> Thank you Jair, for all your help. I went to the Rathaus (city hall) and then to Dr. Quentin. I think I will let the issue drop. I found many websites on my own and have read and learned a lot! I foresee no changes being made because of the financial climate. There is a meeting in the village on March 7th regarding the masts radiation issue, in case you are interested.
> May God bless us all with good health. Thank you for your help. Anne

The following day I decided to see what the small antenna sticking out of that neighbor's back yard was all about. I could see only the back yard from our home. I grabbed my diary showing my symptoms/date/times, and walked around the block and introduced myself to that neighbor. Herr Staubach was a nice gentleman who spoke English— luckily. His wife did not. I explained whom I was, where we lived and that I was feeling ill. I showed him my diary and at first he did not understand and I got no reaction. Then he blanched and pointed to a couple of dates and times and his mouth fell open. He took me into another room, the one that held a ham radio and all his equipment and logs. He went to the top log where he records all transmissions. There he showed me how his dates and mine correlated. On a couple of those dates I had written down symptoms, and the times matched his exactly. The big storm we had experienced had knocked out his antenna. During the storm Herr Staubach had run outside and tried to fix his antenna as best he could. He had wired it incorrectly, giving it too much energy. The regulating federal agency called him the following day and told him to go out and fix the problem as they were getting illegal readings. He fixed the problem. That was the story. While there in his home, I did not feel ill. More, I did not believe his ham radio was making me ill.

>Feb. 5, 2007- email:
>Hi Jair:
>The email address and name you supplied do not belong to anyone that has a mast on the barn, but to a nice little elderly couple at the end of the street with ham radios (amateur radio) and a small antenna in their backyard. After speaking with them for some time, I don't think this is the problem.
>
>Feb. 5, 2007- email:
>Dear Jair:
>This is not a fight one can win. In this case we would be fighting an odorless, invisible enemy that has money. Unless there are dire health problems directly associated with these towers and they are documented, there will be no change. My poor health symptoms might be attributable to other causes. I am bowing out for now. There is too much money invested in these masts, by large corporations such as Vodaphone, Nokia, Motorola, Sony, Siemens and maybe, too, government kickbacks and taxes. I believe this is just the beginning of the airwaves health danger situation. Probably the best thing to do is buy stock in products that would protect people, i.e. fear-based stock, (paints and building supplies made to shield from energy rays) and wait until science and medicine catch up with the reality of people being afflicted with ill health. Until then, pray.
>
>Thank you for your help. Warm Regards, Anne

Anne Mills

Diary-
Feb 1,2007, 11:00PM to1:19AM, into morning: Loud humming. Lots of energy. Lots of pain. No sleep. Tonight rated "5" in strength

Feb 5, 2007, 11:00PM, feeling ill, all night, nauseated, night sweats, to 7AM. Strength "7"

Feb 5, 2007, contacted neighbor, Mr. Walter Staubach, regarding the masts (humming) changes I had heard. DI2AG@fen-net.de oder DJ2LF@Darc.de oder walter.staubach@fen-net.de 09134-7568 http://home.arcor.de/wkhn/html/di2ag_440_khz.html is his old site of 6/2006.

Feb 7, 2007- I'm thinking with the microwave masts, that the phones over here probably wouldn't be used in the middle of the night. I am at a loss as to what else it might be. Went and met with the neighbor, a Mr. Staubach, who had a large antenna in his back yard. What he showed me was radios. Don't know if a radio would do it. He deals in ham radio. He is a cute old guy in his late 70s that used Morse code during the war. I am going to start diary entries to see if I feel it more in the wet weather. Like fighting an invisible enemy. Oh, and Eric and I are moving to a new home. We just need to find the right one.

Feb 8, 2007- During day – Lots of frequency changes – on 10 minutes, off 10 or 20 minutes, on, off, on, off.

Per information I've read, and in speaking with our neighbor, it seems I am having a problem with radiation given off by the cell tower masts. Electromagnetic sensitivity. I believe I am sensitive to something that I can't see. I hear incessant humming, not always at same frequency, at differing oscillations, depending on the night. This happens at night from

11PM to 7AM. I also feel charged or amped up and I don't like it. There are three electromagnetic mast towers on the barn across the field (177 meters) away from us. I feel like we are being beamed, or fried. It is really bothering me and there is little I can do about it. No one here speaks out on his or her own behalf. I think they are afraid of something. The few close neighbors I have spoken to about the problem don't hear, feel, or admit to anything. It's just me I guess. It can only get better, right?

House Shopping
     I am looking for another house closer to where Eric has been transferred and am experiencing a language barrier. I don't know what the newspaper ads are saying. When I call and I speak the little bit of Deutsch I do know, they go on a mile a minute in Deutsche and I'm lost. I have to come right out and ask if they speak English. Much more difficult for me to communicate over the phone than in person, as I find some just hang up, others know a little English and try.

It is time to do taxes, and I must file in both US and Germany. This sounds fun!!

Diary- I am just going into town to do banking, but I could disappear. I am from California, no one knows me here in Germany. My Deutsch is passable. I could run away. It would be so easy. I am already at a bus stop on the way to the train depot. I have my backpack, I am dressed for the weather, I have money, and no one is expecting me. I am one hour from the Czech border, two from the French border and three from Italy. I have eight hours before anyone would find me missing. In eight hours, I could be anywhere. I could run away. I have many things I am tired of facing. But, I have a husband I love. I guess I will think about running away tomorrow, probably while sitting here waiting for the bus.

Feb. 15, 2007 email:
Hi Eric,
I miss you so much. I am alone all day long. If I was closer, as in, we lived closer, would you come home for lunch?
Love Annie

Hi Annie,
Yes, we will make this move happen. I'm sorry that you are alone.
Love Eric

Diary Feb 26- Frequency changed at 2:19 AM instead of 1:19 AM. Every night I feel like I have the flu.

I have errands to attend to in Erlangen, so I am at the little bus stop again. How many times do I think about just disappearing? There are so many things I have to face that it's overwhelming. It's a constant job to keep myself in check, to not just break down and cry. I have no one to talk to, no one to ask for help. I am a California native, living in Germany for my husband's employment. My *job* here, as I see it, is to support Eric. To make a home he returns to, complete with good meals and good company. But my job means that I also do all the finances. This is not always the easiest in a country you are familiar with, but here in Germany, I had to learn how to read a bill. Due to our decision to move closer to Eric's job, I have to find a different house. This means reading and answering ads in the paper and speaking with property agents, in an unfamiliar language, over the phone. The oil tank in the basement of the rental house leaked and stunk to high heaven, and the house hasn't had hot water for two days. Our taxes are due, not only in Germany, but in California, and Eric's employer has submitted our income incorrectly. I just learned that our son is getting married, and I have to plan the flights, gifts and reception dinner. I have to pack the house for the move. This is on top of the grocery shopping I do on the bicycle as we only have the one auto, and banking in a foreign country. Shopping is difficult when no product is familiar and I can't read the label on a bottle. How do I buy meat in grams? Doing the recycling should be simple, but here this is a big job of washing and dividing garbage into seventeen different classifications. Moving includes de-registering in the county, and re-registering in the new county, which meant going to the Rathaus in both places. This means re-registering our autos, at a German DMV, and changing all utilities and insurance policies. I've taken too much on considering I am not feeling well. We believe we are being poisoned with man-made pulsed microwave radiation from the cell tower masts on the barn across the field from our home. It is like having the flu 24/7. I am on max overload. I want to run away. Take deep breaths. It can only get better. Weird, but I have a sudden flashback, of a feeling I had been having in California, as if I had my toes curled over the edge of a cliff. I was standing on the edge. This was about a week before Siemens asked Eric to move to Germany.

Dr. Quentin sent me a Flyer for the local meeting regarding the "MobilFunkSender", or cell towers.

> Weitere Mobilfunksender sind auch in Ihrer Nachbarschaft geplant!!
> Wie Gefahrlich ist Mobilfunk wirklich?
> Offentlich informationsveranstaltung am
> 07 March 2007 @ 19 Uhr 30
> Kolping-Haus Neunkirchen/Brand
> Zugang neben dem Gasthof Zur Post od. uber Kirchplatz ...

I feel like this meeting has been a long time in coming, and look forward to some answers.

March 2, 2007 email to family:

We live by some Electromagnetic Frequency (EMF) radiation-producing cell tower masts that are messing with my health. You know how everyone loves his or her cell phone? Well, cell phones communicate only through cell tower "masts", and those work with, you guessed it, radiation, and radiation seems to be making me ill.

We went to look at a house in Sophienthal (Sofee-EN-thal) we are interested in renting. We really like the new little house, and the listing agent handed us a standard contract and we shook hands with the owner, Heidi—a gentlewoman's agreement. Heidi was nice enough to bring her daughter to translate for us. The house has a nice garden, patios, two garages, small floor plan and no close neighbors. There will be more money outlay than we had anticipated, as we must fill the oil tanks in the basement. Also, we must pay the current tenant back for the flooring she put in, linoleum and rugs. That is how it is done here. We are excited on the way home, talking of the new house and plans.

The new house is available on May 1. We need to be out of our Dormitz house by June 1. Perfect timing. In Sophienthal, there are about four streets and about forty old German houses, but we all share one street name. We are in 6A house, right between 38 and 62. The houses were numbered in order of being built. There is no bakery, meat market, or post office, but there is one cute little gasthaus, or pub/restaurant. Looks like the party is at our house because—we live at the park! Really, the ParkPlatz! We even have our own zip line! Love and Miss you. Anne

Diary
Mar 5, Slept great last night.

Mar 6, Slept terrible, even though I was tired. Woke to being wet from night sweats.

Mar 7, Slept great, then felt more energy, then heard humming, then moved to basement.

The long awaited meeting is finally here:

<u>EMF Electrosmog Meeting</u> In Dormitz Mar. 07, 2007
    Getting dressed takes a while when we aren't feeling well. I am so achy. The bad rashes and welts I've lately developed on the front of my legs itch badly. It hurts to walk and my stomach does not want food. I get my bicycle out of the garage and coast down to the village. Not fun coasting on cobblestones with a headache. Today there is to be a locals meeting about a local cell phone tower, and though it will be in Deutsche, I am going to see if someone, anyone, knows enough English for me to convey what is going on. I am better with charades than Deutsche, but there is no gesture that would convey the weird pain and shaking convulsions that come on a timed basis out of a dark nowhere. Maybe today I will finally get answers.
    The town hall is filled with about one hundred people in various forms of country attire. At the front of the room, by the podium, stand seven tall men in suits, and I can only surmise that they are the experts. I sit through the meeting, not understanding a thing, and only approach the speakers once the meeting is over.
    I feel very out of place, and being barely 5 feet tall, overwhelmed, as I approach and stand in the middle of these tall men in suits. "*Sprechen sie English? Sprechen sie English, Bitte?*" I ask. One of the gentlemen steps from the crowd and in

a very thick accent tells me he speaks English. I feel so lucky. He introduces himself as Herr Peter Wenz, an environmental auditor and researcher. Herr Wenz and I sit and I try to figure out where to begin and what is important and finally decide to just start at the beginning. This means I must cram information that would fill a pamphlet into the size of a business card, but I am taking the only chance I have been given. As it is such a relief to tell anyone, it just gushes out, maybe too quickly for our language barrier, But Herr Wenz gets the gist ... "ringing ears, rashes, hot flashes, nausea, bleeding ears, hair loss, stopped menses, insomnia, and shaking." Herr Wenz stops me, eyes wide, seemingly worried. He tells me these are all symptoms he has heard before and he would be interested in speaking with me further. He says we must talk more and he must see where we live. He gives me his phone number. I give him our address and leave. I don't know much more than I did when I came, but it feels great having had someone listen who maybe knows how to end this horror. Adrenalin makes my bicycle ride to the top of the hill so easy that I don't remember the trip, and amazingly I can eat. The high holds through my telling Eric the good news, but it does not make that night go any better, and once again, for six hours, I shake in pain and confusion.

Diary-
March 8, 2007, Masts on High / Loud / nausea and night sweats "5"

Mar 9, Masts on High / Loud / In so much pain / Grids in morning "7"

Mar 10. Masts on High/Loud / pain and tremors / Grids in morning "7"

March 11, Masts on High Energy – Felt ill all night, night sweats/ grids "8"

Mar 12, Masts Loud and High Energy /all night / pain, pain, pain "8"

I went to the Rathaus in Dormitz to tell the mayor we were leaving and they gave me a form that Eric must sign to leave the county. I am so tired. Next I went to the doctor's office and got copies of my medical records. I then went to the Post to pay property tax for our California house, then to the bank to pay auto insurance and the listing agent. I next went to the market and got a big piece of chocolate cake for lunch. Then to do laundry, realizing I had left the little black hat I've loved for ten years on the bus.

Diary- Mar 12, 2007, Eric and I have been sleeping in the keller for the last month. It's very uncomfortable as the cold comes up from the ground. Those masts across the field, that we didn't notice when we first moved in, are still bothering me. Hear them turn on, change frequency - feel the change - get headaches and nosebleeds and the jitters. Ears bothering me like I talked on the phone for ten hours. For that reason, glad we are moving. And, I really don't need to rattle around in a house this big.

Diary- Mar 13, Turbo-power energy on at 1:19AM. More energy felt—last night terrible –different frequency, not as much energy. I'll give it a "9" and would hate to feel 10. Grids on eyelids in morning, And today at 11AM ON HIGH: bad headache/teeth ache.

Diary- Mar 15, Last night hum not as bad but it did wake me. Only a "4".

Diary- Mar 17, 2007, Rough Night. Last night was a rough night for sleep. The masts have been making me ill for some time now and they make sleep impossible, what with the ringing, humming, ear ache. I can feel when the EMF's (ElectroMagnetic

Anne Mills

Frequencies) change, even though people say no one can. I can! I can feel when the frequency changes, when the power increases, when it goes off. Last night I moved my blanket into the entryway and slept on the floor. Eric has been sleeping in the basement with me because some nights I can feel it a little less down there. Unless they turn up the energy instead of the frequency, and then it is worse being down there. I can't stop shaking—like the jitters.

I am really counting down the days to when we move. The new house is located in a little valley where we will be lucky to get computer at all, and hopefully won't get all the EMFs the house we are in now absorbs. I am sure it will have its own problems, as it seems nothing comes easy to us, but at least it will get me away from these masts. Per what I understood from Peter Wenz, I think the mast that really bothers me is the 3G Mast for computer output. All this is right across the field, not 200 yards from our house. The 3G mast wasn't connected, per the Rathaus, until August or September.

Diary- Mar 20, 07, The masts and the EMF emissions continue driving me nuts: no sleep, headaches.

So, I am packing for the move to the new home. I guess like everything else, one step at a time, one room at a time, one box at a time. Even that seems too much. Just fill the box and set it in the middle of the floor. Luckily, just the sight of an open empty box elicits my packing, and in response, I put together another box. "Let's try one more box." In this way, I take baby steps amid hyperventilating, one room at a time, one box at a time. Take a minute to look at the snow and relax. On to next box. My hands are black with newspaper print. Hopefully, this illness will settle down. I need to take a day or two and mourn the changes and the losses. I haven't done that.

Diary- Mar 23, 07, Looking forward to moving, as the EMFs are really bad. Our winter car broke yesterday and I was so mad at Eric making me be the one to limp it into town and have it fixed today that I spent money on myself. That is what it takes for me to buy myself something. I have to be pissed or feel unappreciated.

On April 17, 2007, I called and spoke with Herr Wenz. He is the researcher that I met at the town meeting regarding cell tower masts. He said he would come over on Thursday or Friday around 4PM to talk and see about setting up some measuring equipment. I told him that when the humming wakes me up, I see grids with elliptical circles in patterns. He said I'm not the first one he's spoken to who has said this. I told him about the physical pain I experience. He told me that when he measured his house he got no signal, but he lives quite a bit farther away, and in a little valley. He said that last month the humming woke him up and he slept poorly.

I told him he had only about a week to do the measuring as we are moving.

Picture: These masts were just across a farmer's field from our house, 170 meters away.

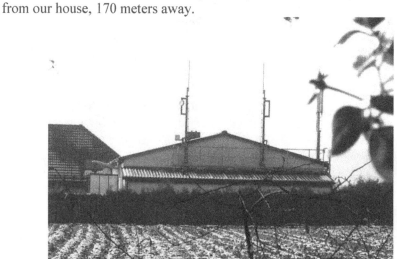

Diary- April 2007, Dormitz house
We have a warm day, and as I walk barefoot on the back lawn, raised bumps reveal acorns hidden beneath the moss and grass. I hate to pull them as I'd like them all to become trees, but then the lawn would look like it did last July, mainly Oak sprouts and mushrooms. Really not much lawn at all.
I have raked piles of leaves from under the bushes where I pushed them off the lawn last fall. The leaf blanket kept the plant roots from freezing, but now they must be removed so that the spring rains can reach the soil. I now push the leaves onto an old sheet that I will drag to a field berm where they can finish decomposing. My fingernails are black with dirt and remind me that since I could walk I've been gardening, and that gardening is comforting to me. Pulling weeds, aerating soil, and watching bugs: a huge part of my life. These too few moments help me ground my soul for upcoming onslaughts of present day madness. Once again I must steel myself from the ever- present

lurking of contemplation. There is too much going on right now to give over to sadness or self-pity. When this is all over, I'll allow this Annie girl a good cry. Right now I must keep myself busy with the mundane. I Love you Annie.

ElectroMagnetic Frequency Radiation Testing
The first time

By this time, my symptoms were much worse. I started getting terrible headaches where before I'd never experienced more than one headache a year. I was losing my vocabulary. I was losing my ability to concentrate. I was losing my motor skills and starting to stumble. I had nausea twenty-four hours a day. I could never get enough sleep.

I walked next door to Jair's house one day, but did not make it. For some reason my body collapsed, as if my bones got soft, and I lost control. My ragdoll body was in the driveway and my head on the curb of the neighbor's lawn. I lay there, scared and aware, but unable to do anything. I am so glad it was late in the day. It felt like I waited forever for help, and I cried when I saw Eric drive up to the house, home from work. He saw me and helped me into the house. He was so mad. Mad at the circumstances that would put us in this situation. He was ready to break contract and go home to California. I was just glad it was not raining or snowing or super cold. I was so glad he found me. I was able to be ambulatory in about half an hour's time, but just knowing this could happen filled me with alarm.

At night when the humming started, I also started to shake from head to toe, as if I was freezing cold, but I wasn't. I just shook. I would walk around the house and try to sleep in different rooms, behind the stairwell, in the bathtub, and again in the car. I was still seeing grids behind my eyelids. I felt driven to get away from the feelings and noise. I was very ill, scared and alone. I felt I was dying. I felt cooked and nauseated.

I asked Herr Wenz to our home to measure, and he came one afternoon with his "calibrated" equipment. He said that his measurements showed "normal" daytime use with small spikes of cell phone usage. He told me that the "medical community has sanctioned "1" as being safe. The government has sanctioned "9 to 15" as being legal. Fifteen is the reading that the research scientists quote as causing rapid changes to DNA. The microwave towers, specifically 3G, use a very low frequency, which is on the same line as DNA. This is what makes it so dangerous. The frequency can cause changes to your and your children's DNA and can cause cancers."

I told Herr Wenz that the masts were not really coming on until nighttime. I said, "But it is not on now. I can feel it when it is on, and it is not on now." I told him that the really heavy humming didn't start until sometimes 2 AM. Peter was amazed that I could "feel" the energy, but politely told me to call him, any hour of day or night. He gave us his phone number, with instructions to call him when the "feeling" was ON.

On the night of April 21, 2007, early morning, at 2:00 AM, I called Herr Peter Wenz, apologizing to his wife when she answered the phone. I told him that the energy was an "8" in my own scale of 1 to 10. A short while later Herre Wenz was at our house and setting up the computer equipment in our backyard. It was a cold April morning, still dark. I was in my pajamas with a blanket around my shoulders as he read his radiation meter. He said, "The meter is showing so high a number that I can't read it. Let me put on a filter." He screwed in a filter of 10,000. The energy was still so high he could not read it. He screwed in another filter of 10,000. Finally, the meter read "7". He was astounded: 70,000. Herr Wenz did a couple more readings. He said that if he was in the laboratory, he'd have to be wearing a "bee suit" for protection, the energy was so high. He told us not to spend another night in the house. Due to the readings, this was going to have to be reported to the German court system.

Herr Wenz also gave us the name and phone number of a physician, Dr. Horst Eger, who was familiar with electromagnetic hypersensitivity. We called and made an appointment to see Dr. Eger.

We moved out of the house the following day.

On the night of April 21, we spent the night above the little bar in Dormitz. Per Herr Wenz' instructions, we did not spend another night in the house. I still felt it when the masts came on. This morning Eric left the rented room for home so he could get ready for work. I stayed and slept for a couple of hours then walked home. We had not slept well. Face it, not only strange bed, but we were above a bar looking out to the street with a neon sign just outside!

I contacted Herr Wenz and told him that Eric would like to help him get the regulations for masts changed. I asked him for a copy of the report and readings he took of the mast. I emailed Herr Wenz a personal letter from Eric and I to be forwarded to the Germany Embassy with his report/readings. He phoned shortly and said he had contacted the German authorities and the Embassy, giving them our letter and the report.

Report – Translated from Deutsche
    European Standardizing Committee Panel of the
    European Commission Medical Devices Auditor LGA and
    Environment Auditor TÜV
    This report consists of the following 5 paragraphs (1) to
    (5)and the additional information ( ) to ( )

Task Settings

A clarification as to the level of the high frequency radiation at the home site of the Mills` family has been carried out due to order. This home site is situated in visible contact to a telecommunication site (Transponder Masts). Ms. Mills is complaining of health disturbances beyond all bearing with no obvious source at all and receives medical attendance.

Mills 20 Apr 2007 Executive Summary

The measuring detected radio link system signals at the home site Mills and within the site building. These signals could be localized and allocated to the telecommunication sites/ Base Transceiver Stations Dormitz/ Schlesier Strasse, Uttenreuth/ Weinberg and Neunkirchen/ Brauerei Vasold.

The level of these signals was detected at a minimum of 20 Watts per square meter. This situation qualifies an acute hazard to health and needs immediate clarification and remedy.

In terms of any liable follow up to the generated results there has to take place the formal notification of the authorities as the federal network authority (Bundesnetzagentur), the district public health department (locales Gesundheitsamt), the federal authority for the protection of radiation (Bundesamt für Strahlenschutz) and the district public prosecution authority Forchheim (Staatsanwaltschaft am Amtsgericht Forchheim).

Ms Mills has been able to detect the time patterns related to the highest radiation levels by her sense definitively, as she has been able to call for the scrutinizing measuring when just feeling the impact of the highest radiation level. The patterns told by Ms Mills have to be conceded as true.

Mills 20 Apr 2007 Protocol
Equipment (1) HF Analyser GS

0,8 GHz/3,3 GHz- 60 dBm resolution minimal calibrated 6 dB

Seite 1 von 5
Third Party Referee EOQ
European Standardizing Committee Panel of the European Commission Medical Devices Auditor LGA and Environment Auditor TÜV cascadable
(2) Log Per Antenna GS directive 0,8 GHz - 2,7 GHz compensated/ calibrated, cascadable
(3) Log Per Antenne LAT very narrow directive GS, not compensated
(4) Attenuation GS 20 dB calibrated, cascadable
(5) Filter GS 20 dB attenuation calibrated 0,4 Ghz - 3,3 GHz adjustable, cascadable
Measuring site Mansion DE 91077 Dormitz / Family Eric u. Anne Mills
Situation overview
Topography Measuring site and all Base Transceiver Stations are apparently on the same ground level.
No verification in the context of this report.
Individual circumstances apparently solid built mansion, ground floor and first floor situated near top of the hill, slightly sub-hill, topmost hill point to the north-west, terrace south,

Seite 2 von 5
Uttenreuth / Dormitz / Neunkirchen / Meßstelle / Norden
European Standardizing Committee Panel of the European Commission Medical Devices
Auditor LGA and Environment Auditor TÜV
Entrance east, garages slightly lower east, spherical hill site, going down north-east BTS Dormitz Schlesier Strasse, distance 150 m level, visible no obstacles to the west north-west 1 plus 2 more buildings (mansions,

homesteads) to the east north-east village buildings. lower ground level to the south south-east buildings front at same ground, level, arranged behind is village at lower ground level southbound no obstacles until BTS
Measuring Setup Signal Strength

Friday 20. April 07 17:00 - 18:30 Uhr (05:00-06:30 p.m.)
particular time with statistically firm high traffic/ high radiation levels.
Basic survey, peak at terrace southbound, basic survey garages, basic survey inside building.
(1,2,4) Level outdoor Min. 10.000 µW/m2
Max. 30.000µW/m2
(1,2,4) Level indoor ground/ first floor
Min. 6.000µW/m² Max. 27.000µW/m²
(1,2,4) Level indoor basement
Min. 500 µW/m² Max. 3.000 µW/m²

Saturday 21. April 2007 03:00 - 03:45 Uhr (03:00-03:45 a.m.)
particular time with statistically firm low traffic/ low radiation levels.
Basic measuring only terrace/ garages in analogy to Friday levels (1,2,4) Level outdoor
Min. 15.000 µW/m² Max. 70.000 µW/m²

Monday 23. April 2007 02:15 - 03:00 Uhr (02:15-03:00 a.m.)
Particular time with statistically very low traffic/ very low radiation levels
Basic Measuring produces very high levels.
Measuring frequency selected with high attenuation.
(1,2,4,5) Level outdoor
0.9 Ghz direction BTS
Neunkirchen

no discrete values
(3.000.000 µW/m²)
0.9 Ghz direction BTS
Dormitz
no discrete values
(3.000.000 µW/m²)
0.9 Ghz direction BTS
Uttenreuth
no discrete values
(5.000.000 µW/m²)
1.8 GHz direction BTS
Neunkirchen
no discrete values
(10.000.000 µW/m²)
1.8 GHz direction BTS
Dormitz
no discrete values
(12.000.000 µW/m²)
1.8 GHz direction
BTS Uttenreuth
no discrete values
(14.000.000 µW/m²)

Seite 3 von 5
Referee EOQ
European Standardizing Committee Panel of the
European Commission Medical Devices Auditor LGA and
Environment Auditor TÜV
2.0 GHz directions BTS
Dormitz as well / Neunkirchen as well / Uttenreuth no
discrete values
(11.000.000 µW/m²)
1.5 GHz direction BTS
Neunkirchen
no discrete values
minimal 20.000.000 µW/m² (20 watt per square meter)

1.5 GHz direction BTS
Dormitz
no discrete values
minimal 20.000.000 µW/m² (20 watt per square meter)
1.5 GHz direction BTS
Uttenreuth
no discrete values
minimal 20.000.000 µW/m² (20 watt per square meter)
(1,2,4,5)
and (1,3,4,5)
Peak results despite maximal attenuation at any one
time in directions BTS Dormitz, Uttenreuth, Neunkirchen
always 1.5 GHz

Mills 20 Apr 2007 Evaluation

At first and taken in account the overall conditions of the
site there has been to assume high radiation exposures.
The time of the Friday setup has been chosen deliberately,
as to ensure statistically firm high radiation levels. The
result of a non-selective accumulating measuring has been
expected within the upper part of the legal limits.

The effective measuring (Friday) results in considerable
lower levels. A likewise nonselective accumulating
measuring has ascertained adequate the buildings
attenuation.

The follow up measuring results have not been in
accordance with the assumed values, given the statistically
data transfer traffic of the BTSs.

Undoubtfully Ms Mills has been able to time the radiation
exposure levels. Ms Mills told time patterns of the
radiation levels can therefore be used for the radiation
source investigation without any doubt.

As to the over-modulating measuring situation on Monday
23. April 2007 there have taken place thorough
consultations with the measurement equipment

manufacturer, which arrives in the conclusion, that the equipment calibration must be conceded valid
with integrity of data results, i.e. peak at radio link system frequency 1.5 GHz.
Overmodulation is due to measurement specifications and starts at radiation levels over 20.000.000 µW/m². **The situation on site suggests multiples of these levels.**
To my knowledge the radio link system signal radiation levels are not subject of legal limits due to hazard to health evaluations/ effects on organism/ since these signals are not supposed to touch either civil/public grounds nor people on civil/public grounds.
Inherent to the system there is to assume high antennae gains and related EIRP.
Hazard to health evaluations have led to compulsory legal limits of radiation as published by the federal authorities 26. BImSchV (federal decree for the protection of emissions Vers. 26).
The measuring results of Monday 23. April 2007, exceed these limits by far.
This situation constitutes a bodily injury/ grievous bodily harm by means of prosecution terms.

Seite 4 von 5
European Standardizing Committee Panel of the European Commission Medical Devices Auditor LGA and Environment Auditor TÜV
Mills 20 Apr 2007 City Date Signature Dormitz 24.April 2007
Time patterns, as told by Ms Mills, the radiation „sensed" beginning approximate August 2006, increasing / rising in November/December 2006 most common pattern of the strongest impact: Thursday/Friday/Saturday
approx. 02:00 a.m. /03:00 a.m.

(end of report)

> April 24, 2007 - email:
> Herr Wenz, Can you please forward this letter for us to the Consulate in Munich. I feel extremely ill and we are leaving the area. We do not have time to wait for your report. Thank you so much, Anne.

We wrote a letter to the American Consulate on Apr. 24, 2007, explaining our situation. We introduced ourselves, told them where we lived and why we found ourselves in Germany, and informed them of my medical downfall. We told them of the testing of the cell tower masts, how the local authorities were apprised of the situation. "Herr Wenz felt concern regarding the findings so he spoke with technicians and doctors, and the readings would be going to the Federal Radiation Protection and Health Office. He said that the situation is an "actual immediate danger" to human health and in this situation there is need to act—as soon as possible.

The measurement findings suggested there were problems beyond all measure with the radio link system of the three nearest fixed transmitter station masts; Dormitz, Uttenreuth and Neunkirchen. We told them also that, because the levels are illegal, this is an illegal situation, and that Herr Wenz handed the information to the prosecutor's office. This bad situation was propelled by big money, and we cannot fight them alone. As an American citizen we asked the Consulate to act on our behalf.

Moving and a Diagnosis

April 25 and 26, 2007

We were devastated with the scary news imparted by the radiation readings Herr Wenz took at our home. So many implications run through our minds, but the worst was health. Though we were told not to spend another night in our home, the only good luck was that we had already planned to move. Most of our possessions were already boxed and in our new landlord's garage a few blocks from the new house. But, we had to quickly find another place to stay for a while, as our new rental closer to Eric's work, would not be available for another two weeks. Wenz helped us find a small apartment in Etlaswind, a little valley, but on the first night I had problems. Eric, in taking a walk the following morning, came across a very close cell phone tower with an antenna cone a short distance away. Eric took time off from work to care for me, as I was too weak to even make myself something to eat.

We needed to move again, and filled the remainder of this day and the following getting everything out of the old rental home, boxed, housecleaned and painted. For the short-term stay we chose a small hotel in the same town as our new home, in Sophienthal. In this way we make the commute easier on Eric, and I could take small walks to get to feeling better and get to know the neighborhood.

April 27, 2007

Herr Wenz contacted us and suggested more readings at the home in Dormitz. He had obtained a more sophisticated computer based spectrum analyzer, a kind of oscilloscope that would not max out. It was the type of equipment used by telecommunications companies in Germany. Eric and I agreed that Herr Wenz would repeat the measuring that weekend, which ensured the report would be very detailed for the authorities.

Dr. Heinlein of Coberg

A couple of days later, Herr Wenz called with the referral of a doctor in the city of Coburn: <u>Dr. Gard Heinlein</u>. He was the Chief of Physicians at the hospital there and had experience with microwave poisoning.

Dr. Heinlein was nice enough to see us after his workday, at 6:00 PM. He told us about his own personal experience with man-made pulsed microwave radiation. He told us that his twelve-year-old son was a very good student, good at sports, and enjoyed an active social life. Suddenly his son was getting in trouble at school, his grades were failing, he was depressed, fatigued, and stopped seeing his friends. Being the chief physician at the hospital, he ran a full battery of tests and they showed some small abnormalities but nothing to point to as a problem. One of Dr. Heinlein's constituents asked him if he had done a timeline about what had changed in the household during that time. In thinking about it, Dr. Heinlein realized that for their son's birthday, they had given him a cordless phone and that he kept it on his nightstand. Dr. Heinlein removed the phone and within a couple of days, his son was back. His son was once again better at school, sports, and socially active. Dr. Heinlein was convinced that electromagnetic frequencies, or EMFs, which cell phone and wireless devices emit, had affected his son's well-being.

Dr. Heinlein read the copies of the reports Herr Wenz had supplied detailing his readings of EMF radiation at our house. He then spoke to us about our symptoms. He had never seen readings so high. I wanted him to explain what the EMFs took out of our bodies and suggest supplements to replace them. I was expecting he would recommend tests with periodic updates. I was hoping Dr. Heinlein would tell us that it would all go away if we took care of ourselves. Instead, he said to get out and stay out of the house. He said that most of the symptoms would go away in a month or so. He suggested we keep a lookout for cancers. Dr. Heinlein said "All I can tell you is to do what you enjoy most." That was scary. To me that sounded like a death sentence, with no hope, and that we should just enjoy life while we had it.

Apr. 28. 2007 - Well, we are not in Dormitz. But I'm still in so much pain: pelvic, breasts, shoulders and hips mostly, I still hear the masts, if only at about a "7" on the energy scale.

April 28, 2007 email response to Herr Wenz:
> Great! Sure, we would love for you to re-measure the Dormitz house. Whatever you need. The house will be locked up, but you have our permission to enter the property. My situation is slightly better, although even our new home has energy that wakes me up. It looks like what we have to do is apply shielding to our new home. We get the key to the new house on Monday and any time you would like, we would love for you to come to visit, to determine the best spots to sleep.
>
> We were able to see Dr. Heinlein of Coberg and we will share your report with him. One point he did mention was that with the levels of energy that we were exposed to we should seek remedy through the court system. Please advise whatever news you have from your escalation through the regulatory agency.
> Thank you for helping us. Anne

April 30, 2007 Herr Wenz contacted us to let us know that "there was a bad reaction from the **Bundesnetzagatur German Regulatory Agency**, and they are setting up examinations under their own supervision."

We move into our new house May 1st, 2007.

Dr. Horst Eger and Diagnosis

We saw Dr. Horst Eger on the referral from Herr Wenz. Dr. Horst Eger is the lead physician, renown for his study on cell phone towers and their impacts on health in Germany. He was not accepting any more new patients, but he made an exception and saw us during his lunch hour, which then stretched into two hours. He had to stop and see other patients periodically.

Dr. Eger, mid 40s and thin, with a wonderful smile and a great office staff, made us feel welcome. This made it easier to tell him our story and our symptoms.

Every time I tell what happened, even writing this, the experiences are relived and re-experienced. That is why I have procrastinated writing all this down.

We started slowly, prompted by Dr. Egers' questions on family health and past health history. He deemed us healthy, normal individuals, and asked us to start at the beginning. So in our beginning, there was nothing. No awareness that anything was not normal. Nothing to be seen. Nothing to be heard or smelled. No smoke. No fire. No sound. We had no inkling, nothing, until it was too late. But when the questions came for our experiences living by a cell phone tower, the dam of hell we experienced in the last several months exploded.

Everything tragic starts out innocent. This case is no different, but as every case is personal and experienced differently, there are twists and turns that often produce similar result.

I first had my menses stop over a period of three months. No pain, No blood. Okay by me. I found this very freeing. But at the same time, I found that my hair was thinning. I have straight reddish-brown hair to my waist, and it was thinning rapidly. Another symptom was that I could not sleep, and at first just laid in bed, eyes wide open. I put it down to being in a strange country. I got a rash on the front of my legs. Large welts that turned to blisters. This rash was very itchy and painful. The over-the-counter creams did not help, and neither did the creams prescribed by the local doctor. This is the main reason I went to see the local doctor, to be told it was menopause, stress and unaccustomed food. Eric intersects in our discussion with his related health issues and his observations of my illness and experiences. Eric is a little clearer than I am, as I am recalling remembered pain and Eric relates as an observer. Eric is my hero.

I also described the plastic bags that lay at the side of my bed to accommodate suddenly nausea. I get drenching night sweats so severe that I have to get up and change nightshirts and lay down towels several times a night. I had unexplained sudden sharp headaches that might only last five seconds, but could be painful enough to make me wince and draw my head to one side. I would be achy, especially in my shoulders. My ankles were achy like I might have arthritis—when neither siblings, parents, nor grandparents ever experienced arthritis.

I would have hot flashes, as one would in menopause, but I had them at certain times. I could actually know when a hot flash would happen, prepare beforehand and know how long it would last.

I told Dr. Eger about my visit to our neighbor's home, when all of a sudden I lost all control of my muscles and fell to the ground, aware but unable to move.

I recounted how I went from fridge to heater trying to locate sounds that matched the hums I was hearing. I told Dr. Eger about the timed hums and showed him my diaries documenting them: how I hear these hums, give them a name, note when they come on, get worse, peak, then go off, only to start again. I tell him how these hums correlate to the pains and body wracking shakes I get. Then I told him about the grids, that I wake up, after a particularly bad night, and have grids on the backs of my eyelids, that last about ten seconds.

At this point, he suddenly stops taking notes. He closes his notebook. He looks quite upset. He questions me about the grids. He has me draw what I see. He tells us this is something he only sees in "vocational poisonings".

Dr. Eger reads Herr Wenz' report. He asks many questions and writes up a multi-paged report on our case. Dr. Eger now tells us that we have been, that I have been, poisoned by radiation from cell phone towers—by the masts. Dr. Eger tells me that I have Electromagnetic Hyper Sensitivity brought about by that poisoning. This will affect me and the way we live, for the rest of my life. This will affect my health for the rest of my life. Dr. Eger goes on to say that radiation goes through walls. Radiation bounces off walls, is reflective, like light. Radiation is very difficult to get away from. Dr. Eger suggests that Eric build what is called a "Faraday cage". This is a metalized cage that holds it's own resistance to radiation. Dr. Eger instructs Eric how to build it, and of what material.

Dr. Eger then writes out orders for testing (blood, neurological, gynecological, internal) and prescriptions for zinc and something to help me sleep. He passes along the name of a research specialist in the states and one of a US lawyer who fought against the American tobacco lobby and won.

Dr. Eger is part of a coalition of physicians, scientists, and academics who have written thousands of peer-reviewed scientific papers showing the dangers of EMF to human health.

Dr. Horst Eger gave us a diagnosis of Electromagnetic HyperSensitivity (EHS)

It looks like I will be spending time in a Faraday Cage.

May 3, 2007 First Official Regulatory Agency Measurements EMF Testing on Dormitz House

Eric had driven me back to the Dormitz house and then continued on to work. We needed to make sure all items were out of the house and the house was in order. So I checked out the house and waited for those who were to do this second EMF testing. A short time later, a Herr Riffer came and introduced himself. He was with the Fulda office of the Bundesnetzagatur German Regulatory Agency but working in collaboration with the Nuremberg and Bayreuth offices. He said he would be the "chief" orchestrating the radiation readings. I left the house shortly after our meeting and walked to the next little town, knowing I needed to be away from this house and its radiation. I felt a little better now being acquainted with someone in charge.

These radiation measurements, unlike Herr Wenz' readings, which were taken in the middle of the night, were taken during daylight hours. I walked back to the house to find the men from Bundesnetzagentur German Regulatory Agency wrapping up their equipment. They quit the testing job just minutes short of when I told them it would get worse. I told these men that the signal would intensify at 17:00 PM, but they quit at 16:45, saying that they had worked more than their normal workday hours and had to leave. The men would not tell us what their readings were. When I called the regulatory agency a couple days later, they refused to tell us what the readings were.

Awareness:

We were now well aware of cell towers and their dangers, but warnings from our meeting with Dr. Heilein, Dr. Eger, and Herr Wenz suggested we should also look around our new home for wireless dangers. Between the experts and our bodies telling us something was not right, our eyes were now open to the effects wireless devices could have. The doctors told us how dangerous our cordless and cell phones were, that even though they weren't in use, they filled our living space with radiation. They told us that Digital Enhanced Cordless Telecommunication (DECT) phones were not allowed in many government buildings or schools. In addition, we had installed Wi-Fi for connecting to the home computer. We had not linked a huge tower and its EMF radiation output to small wireless devices that emit radiation into our home. We had not been aware that, in fact, a cell phone to our head or in our vehicle would still emit radiation. So, we stopped using cell phones, we took out the cordless phone and replaced it with a phone with a cord. We took out the Wi-Fi connection and wired our computer. We stopped poisoning our home environment.

On May 20, 2007, Herr Wenz brought his instruments and measured EMF around the new house in Sophienthal. The area was pretty clear—at least in the afternoon—of microwave energy. He said that we could never get a reading that low in Erlangen. On Dr. Eger's instruction, Eric had built a Faraday cage in the attic. Herr Wenz measured the attic and got a 0 reading: excellent. He said the Faraday shelter was very well made and professional. He told us it was the best we could have gotten had we hired a professional. He said the grounding was fine. There was a debate about whether to ground it as it might act like an antenna. Herr Wenz also checked our neighbor's noisy compressor for EMF and found none, only noise. He did say that if we doubled up on the chicken wire, it would filter out another 90%. He said we ought to be able to shield our bedroom.

It was suggested by one of our doctors that we contact Dr. George Carlo, the attorney who challenged the American tobacco industry. Maybe he would help.

Dr. Eger sent a referral to Dr. Stauch (a neurologist, oncologist, and internist).

Diary: May 30, 2007- Every night we climb a ladder into the attic, where Eric has constructed a Faraday shelter to protect us from the Electromagnetic Frequency (EMF) radiation. I feel caged. Well, I am caged. Our new home is tucked into this little valley at the base of the Fichtelgeburge Mountains. It appears to be an Alpine setting, but like all of Germany, is on a grid of EMF energy. It is all EMF*d Up. At least it is not as severe here as it was in Dormitz. The doctors have said that most of the ill health effects will go away in six to eight months. Due to the poisoning, it was difficult to type or string thought into a sentence. I had lost words and ability to express myself. In order to regain my vocabulary I read many hours a day, trying to concentrate on relearning. We have seen some specialists in the EMF field, but none have treated a condition this severe, so none are prepared to advise us. Instead, they tell us to seek counsel (an attorney).

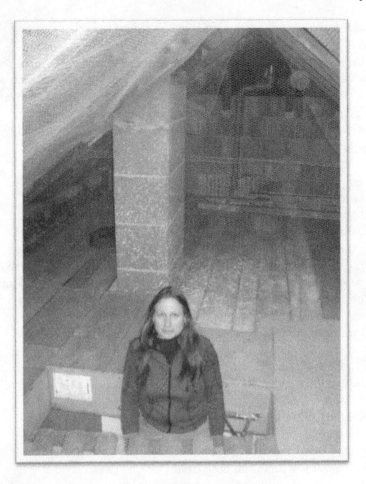

Diary-
June, 2007: I receive an email from Herr Peter Wenz saying he "has agreement with Federal agency...4 nights measuring and this Sunday the manager is going to measure. Yesterday (Wenz) got a call from a doctor who had spoken with Dr. Kleinlein, and

who had run similar tests and who had same results in Coburg area.
There will be an investigation of illegal use of cell tower frequencies and power. He (Wenz) went to the radiation meter equipment company and spoke with the owner. They checked the equipment he used to verify that it is calibrated correctly. Herr Wenz said "There is a situation – unbelievable,...local company <u>not commercial</u> but working with Feds."

Herr Wenz said he had spoken with a government representative for more than two hours. The cell masts were thought to be used for collaborative research between U.S. Defense contractors and their German counterparts.

I spoke with Herr Wenz this morning, June 6, 2007. He has another meeting with Federal officials next week. He told me the company that is doing experiments is "M". "They develop high frequency technological information and modification transmission systems for military and government policymakers (not for commercial use)."
I spoke with Herr Wenz on June 9, 2007, and he said, "that for the last three nights he'd been measuring waves in Dormitz. He measured the highest hill in Dormitz, the one "the church is on and the hill we lived on are each 300% higher in microwave energy than anywhere else." "<u>Like it is a target at a shooting range.</u>" Also, "there is a fourth reading he is getting. He can't figure out where it is coming from."

As the attic is neither heated nor has air conditioning, the temperature there is in constant flux, making it uncomfortable for sleeping in the Faraday cage. For my birthday, Eric built me a new Faraday cage in the bedroom. The bedroom has lovely balcony windows to let in light and air. Eric wired panels, 2' x 5' then wired the separate panels together to form the box. Sadly, this Faraday cage did not work at all. This means I still find myself climbing into the attic Faraday cage. I must wait until it is quite late at night and the attic's sweltering heat has cooled enough for me to sleep.

Today, June 14, 2007, Eric took time off work, driving me to Kronach (kro-Knock) to see Dr. Stauch. She is a doctor of hematology, oncology, and internal medicine referred by Dr. Eger. Dr. Eger had spoken highly of her as a colleague informed about health issues associated with electromagnetic radiation. Her office had a lot of EMF energy and I started feeling nauseous and sore. She took blood tests—ten vials—and so far they have a confirmed a very, very low immune system. She has ordered an MRI and CT scan of my internal organs. Dr. Stauch mentioned that the doctors want to have a meeting, all together, on the issue of my health. Eric then took me to the Apoteke (apothecary) and I got some zinc to help boost my immune system. It was also suggested I take electrolytes.

On June 22, 2007 Herr Wenz called and told me not to do the tests, CT scans and MRI scans, until I am able to bring my immune system up. He must have spoken with Dr. Eger because Dr. Eger called and told me to call Dr. Stauch and that there should be prescriptions there to help me. I called Dr. Stauch and she prescribed three meds. So, I finally had something to bring up my electrolytes, as well as mega zinc tablets. So, finally the doctors have prescribed some medicine—something to try to bring up my suffering immune system. And luckily, I haven't felt nauseated in five days and have had no pain in my ovaries. This is an improvement, but most of the other symptoms are still there. The doctors say it will take six to eight months before I start to feel more my normal self. I can't wait as sleeping in the attic in the Faraday shelter Eric made feels strange. I must climb an attic ladder every night, and climb down to go pee, but this is the only way we can keep the EMF under control.

    I have good days and not-so-good days. The doctors advise me to stay away from stress of any kind—what planet do they live on? We have found someone to translate the radiation reading report. The German sounds scary so I'm not sure I really want to know what it says in English.

Although I have the time, the space, and the equipment to play with art, I have no desire. I don't really care to write. All I want to do is sleep, or maybe sit and weed the yard. Sometimes it is all I can do to make myself a cup of tea. It is scary because I've never been like this. I am turning old before my eyes. Aren't we all, I hear myself saying, but I have lost a good two-thirds of the bulk of my hair! In this new little village where we live there is not much to do during the day, unless I want to go for a walk or ride my bike. It is beautiful here, a narrow valley with forest all around, but even here there are EMFs that I can feel, and it makes me believe that companies have set up EMF energy grids throughout the country.

I have no energy, no spark, and I should be writing. I need to write to some activist groups about this microwave thing going on. Is there a way to change this? I believe that the doctors think I can bring attention to the situation where they cannot because I'm American and I've been injured. I'm the *evidence*. I have to put my "activist hat" on again, but that also means being the aggressor. I've done it several times before in my life. I got all the light poles in our neighborhood newly painted by working with the city parks and roads division. I saved a 200-acre forest from being logged by writing letters to governmental departments and to magazines. I've kept the Dept. of Energy from shipping spent nuclear fuel rods through the town of Concord for storage at the Concord Naval Weapons. I did this by making people aware of the situation we are all in. But this cell tower radiation issue is huge and scary. Where to start? Right now, I don't feel like doing anything but sleeping. I am hoping that the meds and/or electrolytes, something, helps boost my immune system.

I spoke with Herr Wenz on Monday July 2, 2007 and he said, "Feds keep cancelling their meeting. New meeting set for July 13th." He will email over a new report, "once his new readings are taken."

It is almost mid July 2007. I'm feeling better, with more energy and I can now think about more than one thing at a time. I compiled a timeline based on my diary entries of the mast radiation exposures and their intensity and sent it to Dr. Eger and Herr Wenz. I was advised to wait before notifying the ministers and government parties until we have an updated report from Herr Wenz. We should get it soon as the German Regulatory Agency have one last meeting/research mast reading with Herr Wenz this Friday night. That is what Herr Wenz has been waiting for, to finish the updated report. Dr. Eger calls about once a week to see how I am feeling and I feel certain he takes notes.

We have been advised to contact an attorney, but as of yet we have not done so.

I'm starting to have more good days, days when I don't feel I need to go back to bed at 10:00 AM, days when I'm not too sore and have more energy. I've had a couple of days when I can think well, like my brain is waking up. I'm getting my vocabulary back. I haven't had the *nauseous all day* feeling for about two weeks now, which is great. I'm still climbing the ladder into the attic to sleep in the cage. People don't realize how dangerous the 3G and 4G are. And because so much money is invested in this new technology, it will be a long time before anything is done to curb cell tower mast usage. Another problem is that the symptoms of poisoning are not unlike those associated with other, more common, medical problems. The Faraday cage has helped me significantly.

Now I want my sense of wonder and humor back. I feel like I lost a part of myself.

July 14, 2007 – Second Official test by the regulatory agency of our Dormitz house

Eric spent a couple hours with Herr Wenz and about five German Federal administrators at our old home in Dormitz. They were retesting the area for radiation, EMFs. I did not go, instead waited in the car a few blocks away and read a book and slept until Eric called me to pick him up. This was their last test and it was to have lasted until 4:00 AM. They would not tell us the results. I slept well in the car while the testing was being done, so they probably got a very low reading.

A couple days later I called the regulatory agency and asked for the gentleman who had been in charge of the first radiation reading, the chief, Herr Riffer. I was told he had been moved to a new job. Now not being familiar with anyone, we have little recourse. Unlike the previous tests, this time even Herr Wenz has not given us any details. We did not know the time of day they tested, or whether it was more than one day. For some reason, we were being kept out of the loop.

On July 17, 2007, I tried to speak with Herr Wenz regarding the readings, but he would not speak, saying he had been threatened by the German Federal government with losing his job. His wife was also afraid. He "wanted his children to go to a good school. He did not want to move." He "did not want to speak to us on the matter, afraid for his life holdings." Herr Wenz refused to speak of the EMF poisoning and readings.

So, after speaking with Herr Wenz, we contacted a lawyer and were told it would cost millions of dollars to process a lawsuit against a huge corporation that had government backing.

We suspected the company that produced the radiation signals was there in the same town as the towers, Uttenreuth.

That same day, I wrote a letter to the American Consulate chiding them for their lack of concern:

> July 17, 2007
> Hello Ms. Price:
> As American citizens, we wrote a pleading letter on April 24, 2007, asking for assistance with an environmental health problem our family was subjected to here in Germany. We have not heard back from you, the American Consulate.
> We spoke in person with Eric Nelson on July 10th in Bayreuth, and received a form-letter reply suggesting we "get a list of attorneys on our internet site and contact the Green Party." We do not understand why he would suggest the Green Party as they voted against the issue we brought to Eric Nelson's attention: stricter regulations for cell tower masts.
>
> Our problem needs personal attention, thought, and action. Our family has been poisoned by high and illegal levels of electromagnetic radiation frequencies from computer data masts operating with Federal government knowledge. We have research documents confirming said poisonings, showing the illegal radiation levels, a report showing the accuracy of the measuring devices, and confirmation of the Federal government's involvement. Our family now faces years of recovery and the fact that cancers might be inevitable in our future.

Can you help us? We would like a letter stating the
intent of the American Embassy to protect the health of
American citizens. Our next course of action will be
taking this issue to the media.

I have attached a write-up of the issue at hand. When we
see you we will bring the original research papers. We
will be at your conference on Wednesday in Bayreuth,
and look forward to meeting you.
The Mills Family

On July 18, 2007, Eric and I attended the meeting in Bayreuth to introduce ourselves to the vice consulate general from the American Consulate in Munich. The President of the German-American Friendship Circle in Bayreuth was organizing this visit. It was an informal gathering over coffee and cake. We spoke with the vice consulate general, Dr. Lisa Washburn, asking for a letter of support from the Embassy. We had invited Herr Wenz and Dr. Eger, but they were unable to attend.

End of July: Good news. We just got a letter from the Embassy. They want the address of those who have done the testing, and names of those in charge of radiation/microwave poisoning. Their letter states they will send them a letter along with the research papers from Herr Wenz, and the letter we sent the Embassy. We are going to ask for a copy of their letter.

Diary- August 8, 2007, My blood tests came out negative. I think I will be okay. I've slept about six hours the last four nights. Big improvement.

Herr Wenz's first report is now being translated into English. We will get in touch with a lawyer once the first report is translated.

Diary- August 1, 2007, Last night a bad night. Energy on high at 11:00 PM, then higher still in the early morning. Shakes, aches, grids, heart palpitations: not good. "8".

August 13, 2007, We finally receive a letter from the American Consulate stating that they will get involved and are sending a letter along with the report to the German Radiation Regulatory Agency.

We received the translation of the letter from the American Embassy addressed to Herr Riffer of the EMF Regulatory Agency:

>August 14, 2007
>Dear Mr. Riffer:
>The American Consulate General in Munchen is representing the interests of U.S. *Staatsburgern* who live in Bavaria. Family Mills from Weidenburg contacted us. Mrs. Mills has suffered substantial health damage from radiation poisoning the family was exposed to while living in Dormitz, according to a statement of radiation testing.
>
>We are sending you the letter Mr. Mills sent so you can follow up with this affair.
>With friendly greetings, Dr. Lisa Washburn

It is mid August, and as the bedroom Faraday cage doesn't work well, and the attic Faraday cage is either very hot or very cold, Eric built a third new shelter. It is so nice, and much bigger than the bedroom shelter. It is built in the basement, or *keller*, and has both a window and a heater, which the attic did not have. This makes the space light and warm. He double-wired the whole thing but the floor has only one layer. The top of the cage is not touching the keller ceiling. It is very airy and not claustrophobic. We used it last night, and slept very well.

I spoke with Herr Wenz Tuesday, Aug. 21, 2007. He suggested "he might not have received the report from the regulatory agency which was expected about a week ago." He believes it is "because they might have received the letter from the U.S. Embassy and decided to change the report, thus would need more time."

Again Dr. Eger requested more information on EMF radiation readings. I tried once again to speak with Herr Wenz regarding the readings, but he refused to speak of the incident.

Email, Aug 30 2007:
>Hi Eric:
>Is there a way, either at lunch by coming home early, or by leaving work early this evening, that we can run some errands? We need to bring bottles to the *trinkemarkt*, set up for the post to hold mail, and send monies to the States. Also, maybe we should write a letter to the Embassy, telling them that the report from the German Feds was promised in seven to ten days, but upon their receipt of the letter from the Embassy, they suddenly decided to rewrite the report. We are now wondering about cover-ups and untruths surrounding the poisoning. Love, Annie

Sept. 13, 2007, email:
>Hello Dr. Eger:
>I just got a call from Dr. Stauch's office. For some reason, they did not receive the CT scan I took, saying I did not keep the appointment—even though I did. Dr. Stauch did not show up for the scan appointment. The CT was done by the hospital staff who said they were

told not to take an MRI. The office also said they made appointments for me for the other tests, the neurological and breast CT, though I never received dates and times for appointments from their office. I went to the only CT appointment I had, and that was in July. Since that CT scan, my menstrual cycle has not returned. I have not had menstrual bleeding since that CT scan.

We visited California for a week towards the end of September. I have missed my family and friends so much. Eric and I participated in the motorcycle run we started in 1978. This is a yearly gathering where we race up and over Ebbets, Monitor, and Sonora passes with a number of motorcyclist friends. We camp, then race back home. On one of the days, I met with girlfriends and we had lunch. Wow, Mexican food that tastes like Mexican food, and a Margarita with ice! We saunter around town, talk about art and family. I feel normal for a little while. It is difficult to get back on the plane. I don't want to go back to Germany.

Sept. 27, 2007: back in Bavaria. We still have no input from the American Embassy:

I think we need to write to the Embassy again, stating that we have not seen any activity from the German government. We need to bring to the Embassy's attention that Germany's lack of forthright effort to name the known EMF poisoner suggests the impeding of justice and the condoning of unsafe, inhuman and criminal activity. The government's refusal to name the (industry) poisoner points not to the poisoner not being known, but to their being in bed with those same poisoners. The readings confirm that the poisoner scaled back the EMFs being emitted after the testing was done, so if the government was able to ask and have the volume of the tower energy scaled back, then they clearly know who the poisoner is. That is my reasoning, anyway.

We did hear back from the law offices of Peter Angelos. They requested information be returned to them. They also wanted to know who referred us.

Sept. 28, 2007 - I went to see Dr. Eger today, and at his request brought pictures of the old house, the new house, and the Faraday shelters at the new house. We brought along the diary of how I felt in California when we visited. Dr. Eger wanted our translator's email. He will write a report in German and the translator will translate his report. Dr. Eger still wants to do more tests, not to ascertain if there are health effects from the mast energy, but to prove that no other medical condition could have caused the symptoms experienced when the masts were on. They expect to see nothing. So far they have found nothing wrong. Other people have had complete normal activity and health after five or six months. This was nice to learn. They want to prove the masts caused the symptoms and nothing else. This is the medical report he will send to the lawyers.

We mailed off a new letter to the Embassy on Oct. 25, 2007, hoping they will help us get the report from the German government.

Nov. 02, 2007 email:
> Hello Dr. Eger,
> Here is a site that I found that mentions Germany and what it has done in the radiation poisoning field. I send along other areas/sites to contact. Is seems it is time to start telling our story, or do we need to wait for the government to come through with their report?
> Thank you, Anne

Nov. 28, 2007, Received Second letter from American Consulate, and a copy of the letter they sent to the German regulatory agency, Bundesnetzagentur, from the American

Embassy. They didn't forget us. We, however, are puzzled as to it's meaning, and guess that it is to remind the regulatory agency of their responsibility. The letter to the Bundesnetzagentur Regulatory Agency from the Embassy says this:

> "We turned in August to you regarding the family Mills from Sophienthal. Now the Family Mills has asked us again for assistance. Mr. Mills writes that they received notice from your agency that they will not receive a full report until mid September. Unfortunately, the family Mills, to date, has received nothing more from you. We ask again that you follow up directly with Mr. and Mrs. Mills on this issue."

Dec 11, 2007 email:

> Hello Dr. Eger:
> I am having a terrible time sleeping. I have been taking the herbal supplement Balderian as sleeping aid. It no longer works and I lay, hour after hour, trying to hold still so Eric can sleep. I am not falling asleep until about 4:00 AM, and then for only about an hour. Is it possible for you to fax a prescription to my *apoteke* in Weidenberg? Or, do you have any ideas for sleep? Also, although I don't have them during the day, at night I have multiple hot flashes. This does not help my sleep either. My ears ring terribly and only seem to get worse, to a point where it is getting hard to endure the ringing. Thank you for your help. Anne

2008

On Jan 13, 2008, Eric and I travelled back to California for our son's wedding. What an exciting time. Our only child was getting married to a wonderful woman. The bride was beautiful, as was the whole wedding. I had missed my Mom, Dad, and family immensely. I missed the way things used to be and the way I used to feel. I was excited to go, but was afraid that I would not want to get back on the plane to fly back to Germany.

It surprised me that I heard the energy masts humming in California. I thought there wouldn't be any mast radiation there. The masts woke me in the morning, even out of drug-induced sleep, but I didn't suffer the bad pain and discomfort I had in Germany. On packing to come back, I realized that I hadn't had hot flashes since the third day of our visit to California. I'd been having them frequently in Germany and had experienced about fifteen hot flashes on the plane coming to the states. Not a one since that third day! I decided I was going to keep track of how many days it took for them to come back once I returned to Germany.

January 23, 2008 -We were back in our home in Germany. I contacted Dr. Eger several days later and let him know that since our third day back I'd been having night sweats, but didn't have them in California. I realized that while in California I hadn't needed the mid-day nap I did in Germany. I also had more energy there.

Dr. Eger had told me earlier that it might take six to eight months for most of my symptoms to go away.

Diary- Jan 25, 2008
Masts came on big-time last night at 1:30 AM. I saw grids, even after my eyes were open: hexagons with dots in the middle with a line between each one—whole pages full, my eyesight full. Some pain in ovaries and breasts and a headache that kept moving around my head, not really in one place. I haven't had this before, but this went away after the masts were turned off. This lasted a couple hours. Pain on "7" scale.

In early February 2008, Eric and I ate dinner in Bayreuth, sitting next to a gentleman who was a retired high-ranking official in the German government. He told us that he had travelled extensively for the government. Upon telling him our EMF poisoning story, he suggested that we contact an attorney for advice and ask the attorney to retrieve the government report on the EMF readings.

Diary- Feb 8, 2008. Slept pretty well in basement keller.

We spoke with a local attorney and she told us that she could not request the names of the mast owners or users from each city, but that we could. She advised us to write a letter to the three cities that have the masts, and request from the burgmeisters (mayors) the names of the owners and users of the masts. I have called the town of Dormitz, and spoken with Herr Weber, who helped me last year. He said he would get me the information. I have yet to write the other burgmeisters as an election is in process and Herr Weber thought it prudent to wait until after the elections are over. Also, the letter will have to be in German, as he thinks they do not speak English.

So, March 10, 2008, as per Dr. Eger suggestion, we contacted Peter Angelos, Attorney at Law in the United States. He is the lawyer I mentioned earlier who fought and won against the tobacco industry. We emailed his office our story, and copies of the EMF radiation reports. Mr. Glenn Mintzer, attorney from that office, wrote back:

Dear Mrs. Mills:
I spoke with both Dr. Eger and Attorney Herr Kran-Zembol last week. Based on review of the information you have provided, <u>we will not represent you</u> or take any action on your or your family's behalf. Please be advised that if you wish to pursue a possible claim any further, you should contact another attorney immediately.
Glenn Mintzer

On March 18, 2008, Dr. Eger called and suggested we contact a German lawyer, Krahn Zembol. Upon telling Herr Krahn Zembol our story and showing him copies of the EMF radiation reports, he told us he would not be able to help. He "didn't want to get involved."

Diary- April 2, 2008, Masts on early morning, 1:00 AM and 3:30 AM. I hear them; I feel them.

Diary, April 3, 2008, Mast on 1:00 AM. & 3:30 AM.

April 4, 2008, Letter from German Regulatory Agency—finally.
    Along with the letter the government report. We paid 500 euros to have it translated, and forwarded a copy to Herr Wenz and Dr. Eger. It said just what everyone thought it would say: Everything is fine.

    After nearly a year, the Bundesnetzagatur German Regulatory Agency commented that they could not replicate the emission readings. They did not even take nighttime readings for over two months after the initial dangerously high readings were reported to them. We were hoping that the regulatory agency was trying to replicate radiation readings taken over multiple days by the trained technician utilizing two different forms of calibrated measuring equipment. We felt frustrated. It appeared they were not in good faith trying to validate the earlier readings at all. We think there was close collaboration between the regulatory agency and the owner they are working to protect, this ringing particularly true given that there were threats of retribution issued against the whistle-blower, Herr Wenz.
    I was in the car, in the area, when the readings were taken that evening, and the energy levels felt very low to me. What we surmised later is that the local antenna/mast company was working in collaboration with the American Defense contractors. Our written complaints and the radiation readings

had been shared with the German Regulatory Agency, which alerted them. They then coordinated their measurements to protect the perpetrators. The German regulatory agency then finally reported back to us that all readings had registered as within permissible limits.

April 22, 2008   Along with the letter from the German regulatory agency and U.S. Consulate we sent the report to Dr. Eger. We also sent a copy of the opinion of the translator.
    Our letter to Dr. Eger:

Hello Dr. Eger,
    We received this opinion from our translator, regarding the governmental report he translated for us. He states rather eloquently, our feelings on the matter, and we wonder if there is someone who can look into this matter further. What are your thoughts? Thank you,
Anne

The translator wrote this:
    On a personal side note regarding the last formula (calculation) and paragraph:
    I am no expert on this matter and it may well be a shot in the dark, but from what I remember from studying biophysics, I know I would start off by looking at the last formula to see how it reflects the fact that different frequencies have different effects on the human body. I would have thought that certain frequency ranges (especially those in the low ghz range) might be weighted higher than other, perhaps less relevant, frequencies. The formula provided in the text does not seem to reflect this, but rather <u>sums up entire ranges instead, thus leading to the effect that damaging effects of certain frequencies are evened out. In my personal opinion, the formula does not necessarily reflect the hazardous effects of electromagnetic radiation as accurately as possible, but rather seems to be a general indicator of the average radiation level as summed up over all frequencies (100khz - 300ghz).</u> But this is just my personal opinion. I think the last formula is something I, personally, would try to get an expert opinion on.

Hello Dr. Eger
Does this mean that the governments report is "averaging" to avoid the true scope of the severity of the radiation readings? Anne

Dr. Eger wrote back:
Thank you for the paper. The (government) measurements were below the level of the measurements Herr Wenz had taken…but the two time points for the measurements were different. So we are told, "everything is alright", because we are within the current limits. I didn't get a copy of the second mast readings, and there has been no further contact by Herr Riffer.

Diary: May 5 thru May 11, 2008, This week, the masts have been on very light pulse and I was able to sleep in our real bed. I felt more mast activity early morning, 5:00 AM, which is unusual.

May 16, 2008
Eric and I travelled to Berlin with Gabe and Uwe (our close neighbors) to visit their mothers. After half an hour on the autobahn I felt very ill.

May 17, 2008, Felt ill on and off all day, bad headache, terrible nausea, and achy, but different symptoms during different blocks of time. I guess Berlin also makes me ill.

May 18, 2008, I feel very achy in shoulders and back, and in my bones. No headache, no nausea. There must be a mast nearby. I get no vacation from EMF.

May 19, 2008, We can't afford to pay for a lawsuit against the German companies, mainly because they have unlimited government access and retain their own attorneys. If this

Anne Mills

becomes a lawsuit, the doctors in this community think we might be able to win, and thus help Germany move toward airwave regulation. We suggest that the community physicians put their money together and pay for a lawyer. This way, before we go back to the States, we can go to court. If we win, the doctors get paid back. This should not be something that is entirely on our shoulders if this might result in healthier environment for German citizens.

<u>*Diary: May 19 to 25, 2008,*</u> *This last week, again, very light energy. Maybe everyone is on vacation. "2"*

<u>*May 26, 2008*</u>*, We are on a two-week motorcycle trip in Italy. Today in Cinque Terre, Felt masts pulsing strongly in the middle of the night. Manarolla: loud ringing and grids, ovary pain, tooth pain, but only on upper jaw. "7"*

<u>*May 27, 2008,*</u> *Same mast energy as yesterday.*

<u>*May 28, 2008*</u>*, In Northern Austria, even though I could see masts a half kilometer away or closer, I did not feel them much. Some ringing in ears, but that is all. "3"*

<u>*May 29, 2008*</u>*, Same mast energy as yesterday and no symptoms.*

<u>*May 30, 2008*</u>*, We are home in Sophienthal, and not much mast energy. Good!*

<u>*May 31, 2008*</u>*, Not much mast energy.*

<u>*June 3, 2008*</u>*, Light. "2"*

<u>*June 4, 2008,*</u> *Light. "2" Masts unusually light the first week of June. I could even sleep in the bedroom. It helps if the door to the balcony is open, as I don't feel reverberations, No pains or*

grids either. I felt more during the day, aches and depression, and fatigue.

June 9, Felt mast at 4:00 AM I had ovary pain, ear ringing, stomach upset (unusual). But no grids.

June 10, Felt masts— woke up at 2:00 AM or so and went to the Faraday cage in keller.

Eric and I went into Bayreuth towards the end of June, and there happened to be a table in the town square with a banner that read "Against Mobile Funk." Those at the table were trying to make passersby aware that it is not only cell phones—in Germany called *handys*—that should concern them, but also the cell tower (mast) that the messaging is sent through. At this booth we met a gentleman named Joachim Weise. Herr Weise works as an environmental analyst and building biologist. He professionally measures EMF for businesses and homes. We spoke with him and he had never heard of radiation poisoning levels as high as the readings that had been recorded at our home. We later sent him a copy of the report by Herr Wenz.

Diary - July 25, 2008, Last night, Eric and I spent the evening at a friend's house here in our little village. Suddenly, starting at 9:00 PM, both of us got a terrible headache. I had a heaviness in one spot of my head and bad ear-ringing and achy shoulders. We left shortly after. Later that night I awoke, still with the bad headache, ear-ringing and achy shoulders. I felt nauseated on and off all night. This was a light energy night compared to most. I woke Eric up to tell him I was going down to spend the rest of the night in the cage. He said he was coming with me because he also felt ill and had a headache. It was so much better in the cage, but we still had a fitful, headachy, nauseated night. Woke right up at 4:00 AM. Don't know why. We got up at 6:00 AM. But, I still have my headache. It is 8:20 AM. This is unusual.

Diary- July 25, 2008, I was told that "the German government might not like the radiation poisoning report getting out, and might end my life sooner than I'd expected." I heard this from those in the "No Mast Mobilfunk" organization. That just amazed me, that anyone would express that, but they must know—they live here. This is getting scary. We must live here in Germany to fulfill the four-year contract Eric has with Siemens. So how much do we fight against the cell tower masts, and are we doing this alone?

July 27, 2008, No Fight Left! Email I sent to Joachim Weise:

> Sorry to disappoint you, but I have decided not to continue to fight. If I can't go the *good* way, meaning through the court system to request an apology and a change in industry regulations, or even compensatory healthcare for the remainder of our years, then I don't want to fight the system. The only way to go through the court system is with monetary help from the German people, or local doctors who want to bring about change. If it is not worth it to them to give monetary help, then I'm not going to, again, put my life on the line. I am not going to *stir the pot* or cause trouble and maybe get myself killed—if I don't have the backing of the people I'm trying to help. It is not worth shortening my life. Do I give the government a black eye when they have a bigger stick, and I don't have Germans to back me up? No. If the community thought I could help, they could back up their ideals with money for an attorney, and a fair fight.

I feel afraid and alone. In California, by myself, I might feel safer, but I have heard from a person that is familiar with this incident, that I could get shot. Sounds far-fetched, yes, but we know personally someone involved in this incident who was threatened with job loss. It's not worth it. The German regulatory agency told me that Herr Riffer, the gentleman who did the first EMF test, was supposedly moved to a different position the day following EMF measurements in Dormitz. I am losing sleep. Anne Mills

> Hello Anne:
> I can understand your position very well. The court system will tell us that the official measurement will be
> the right one and that there are no problems of industry being over the limits. But I will guard your case. I understand and can't blame you. You have got my email address. If there is something new that comes up, please let me know. All the best to you. Joachim Weise

Diary- August 5, 2008, 1:00 AM this morning, masts turned on high. Eric even felt them and woke up. I was in deep sleep and woke up with bad allergies—sudden stuffy nose, itchy throat, itchy eyes, and severe headache. My top teeth hurt and for some reason, unlike symptoms before, and both armpits hurt. We were in the bedroom but we moved down into the Faraday cage in the keller.

After a while most symptoms cleared, but I still felt the high energy and saw mild grids. I slept between the bed and the wall, on floor. I do this about a third of the time.

I had a lung test, an MRI (MRT) and a breast ultrasound. Everything is okay so far.

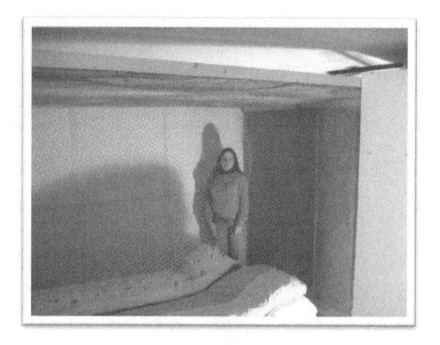

    My Faraday cage is fully enclosed with double wire mesh, including a full-wire door, and ceiling, walls, and flooring. Eric wrapped it with continuous rolled wire, and where the wire walls meet, we sewed them together, in place, with strand wire. One notices a difference once the door is closed. One cannot get cell phone service within this shelter. This is the third one Eric has built in this house. The first was in the attic, the second in our bedroom, and now the third in our keller. We don't use the attic shelter, as the attic is not insulated. We dismantled the bedroom shelter as Eric had tried a different design and it did not seem to work.

All EMF*d Up

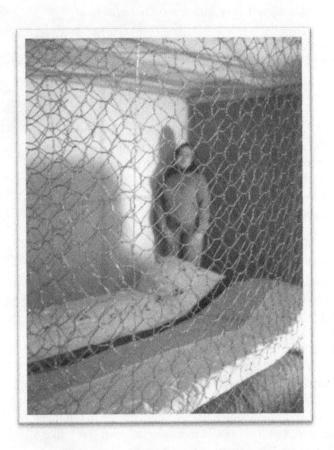

2009

> Dear Annie
> I consider myself very lucky, mostly because of you!!!!!!!
> I'm also feel rich living in the heart of Europe. We are going to have a *Great* year.
> All my love, Eric

I think my husband loves me. Happy New Year!

January 24, 2009 - Per my doctor's suggestion, I had my metal dental fillings replaced. He did not want them to act as antennae, so I had all three of the mercury fillings replaced with porcelain. The dentist used a rubber dam inside my mouth, and a mask over my nose so I wouldn't breathe in the mercury vapors. I was told to take massive doses of Vitamin C and activated charcoal to bind and pass the mercury because it is a carcinogen.

February, 2009 - Eric and I went grocery shopping the other day, and, within just a couple of minutes of walking into the store, I started getting dizzy and disoriented. All thoughts left my head. I forgot what I had come for and lost my vocabulary. I took missteps and had vertigo. I lost confidence and felt unsure of myself. I suggested to Eric that we leave immediately. Eric had gotten a headache right away too. A feeling of confusion, even mistrust of surroundings, left me clutching Eric's sweater for support. We left, but I continued to feel ill for four hours. Not all the stores have WiFi this bad. This does not happen in public as often as it used to, but it served as reminder of what it felt like all the time at home for those many, many months. Very scary.

In March, 2009, I awoke with an incomplete memory of a dream. I recalled horses and a rocky beach. It wasn't so much what the dream was about as it was that it was a dream. I have always had vivid dreams and wrote my dreams in a diary. I have a collection of books explaining dreams. That morning, that dream, woke me to the realization that I had not had dreams in a couple of years. I was amazed that something as important to me as dreaming had vanished. I had been experiencing dreamless sleep. This made me believe that my absence of dreams was another symptom of the EMF poisoning.

June 19, 2009 - I have so many questions, and most of them center around "Why me? Why us?" How could this be legal? Were we just in the wrong place at the wrong time? Were we part of a human experiment or was our poisoning an accident? There is a code called the Nuremberg Code, initiated in Germany at the end of WWII, that offers guidelines regulating human experiments. One of the Nuremberg Code's principles for human experimentation clearly states that the voluntary consent of human subjects is absolutely essential. Would this Code apply in our instance? Because the radiation emitted from the cell towers was so excessive, it makes me believe that I could not possibly be the only one in the neighborhood who became ill.

Moving back to California

> July 02, 2009
> Hello Dr. Eger,
> This is to let you know that Eric has been advised that Siemens needs him back in California. We will be leaving Germany and moving back to California at the end of September, in three months. Thank you so much for all the support. We have enjoyed working with you and your great staff.
> Best Wishes, The Mills Family

It is time to pack once again. It doesn't seem that long ago that we found ourselves packing to start this venture. I approached our friends and acquaintances in the village and asked them if they would like to have our furniture. Siemens contracted for help in this move, so moving men came to help pack. So nice I didn't have to pack alone, and that all our belongings were in the truck in very short order. Wow, moving men! I feel rich! We had said our goodbyes and cried our tears with friends and neighbors, vowing to write often. We dismantled the evidence— our Faraday cages. I was hoping I would never have to sleep in a cage again.

Our life in Germany had been wonderful, despite the EMF radiation poisoning and probable future ill health. I love how clean the streets are and how safe I feel out on my own. Eric and I have shared special times with wonderful new friends. Our new life's dictates took us to The Netherlands, Belgium, Hungary, Scotland, Austria, France, Czech Republic, and to Italy multiple times, in the car and on our sport motorcycle. We will miss Germany's colorful pageants, tractor meets, and beer festivals. It seemed we couldn't turn a corner without a castle coming into view, and we were never one to pass up a castle. Castles were our siren-calls and they took us on unexpected and cherished adventures. But I will not miss the weather. It is time to go home to California weather and family and friends.

Recap*

June 2006, Moved to Germany
Sept-Oct 2006, Health issues began.
Mar. 7, 2007, Electro Smog EMF meeting at local Community Center
Apr. 20, 2007, First EMF Radiation reading of cell tower mast, done by Herr Wenz during daytime hours.
Apr. 21, 2007, Second EMF Radiation reading: Night measurements at 2 AM, done by Wenz. (0200), Herr Wenz told us that the measurements were "so high that were he in the lab doing experiments, he would have to wear his protective bee-suit

body gear. That the "readings were so high, that they would have to go to the court." He was extremely distraught and went straight home to write up his report.

Apr. 22, 2007, Radiation reading equipment/computer checked by manufacturer for accuracy. It was reported to me that the equipment was exact. (calibration check)

Apr. 23, 2007, Third EMF measurement by Herr Wenz

Apr. 25, 2007, We write letter to American Embassy asking for their support.

Apr. 28, 2007, Fourth EMF measure by Herr Wenz

May 01, 2007, Diagnosed with EHS by Dr. Horst Eger

May 03, 2007, First official Regulatory EMF radiation reading: Daytime only

June 1, 2007, Herr Wenz has two hour meeting with Feds-EMF stating to me later that it "was not commercial readings" I understood this to mean that the frequencies and power levels noted were not licensed for wireless communication. I took it to mean that only government had authority for these bandwidths.

June 6, 7, 8, 2007, Fifth, Sixth, Seventh measurements of EMF at Dormitz by Herr Wenz

July 2, 2007, Herr Wenz: "Feds keep cancelling appointments"

July 10, 2007, We speak in person to US Consulate Minister, Eric Nelson.

July 14, 2007, Second official Regulatory EMF measurements: Nighttime.

July 16, 2007, Herr Riffer stops communication. His managers say he is no longer on job.

July 16, 2007, We again write a letter to the US Consulate asking for their help.

July 17, 2007, Herr Wenz threatened by Feds.

July 17, 2007, We are told to contact a lawyer, so we do.

July 18, 2007, We personally speak with Vice Consulate General from Amer. Consulate.

Aug. 13, 2007, First escalation letter from American Consulate to German Regulatory

Anne Mills

Nov 28, 2007, Second escalation letter from American Consulate to German Regulatory
Apr. 3, 2008, Letter from German Regulatory Agency saying in essence "they found no code violations".

    We will probably never know who is responsible for the massive radiation emissions or the purpose they served. We only know their lasting effects. We know that the transmissions were illegal and were reported to the German Court system. We know that the German Regulatory Agency decided to take measurements on its own, once during daytime hours, and two months later at night. We know that the German Regulatory Agency refused to release said measurements. We know that it took three letters from the American Consulate in Germany to get the Regulatory Agency to issue any official response. We know that the German Federal government met with and threatened the research scientist who performed the radiation readings. We were told that the high EMF radiation modulation and energy output would not have been allowed for commercial use. With all the rules and regulatory agencies in Germany, we feel certain the transmissions that harmed our health were known to be excessive. We were told that the "M" (EMF) company in the adjoining town of Uttenreuth works with companies contracted by the American Defense Department. At the same time, we heard talk of German incoming missile defense company called Raytheon.

    When we contacted a lawyer, Peter Angelo, we were told it would cost many millions of dollars to have a lawsuit against a huge corporation that had government backing. Attorney Krahn Zembol, a German lawyer, told us he did not want anything to do with the case.

    We were able to have an expert look at the radiation readings taken at our home in Dormitz: Lloyd Morgan is a senior research fellow at the Environmental Health Trust, a member of the Bioelectromagnetics Society, board member of the

International Electromagnetic Field Alliance, Scientific Advisor of the EM Radiation Research Trust, and author of two legislative acts mandating cancer registry data collection of all brain tumors. He is a published researcher. Upon reading the report (Jan.10, 2019), these were his comments on the radiation readings taken by Herr Wenz:

Radiation measurements: 20 Watts per square meter.
> "This is an astronomical intensity. In the U.S. the maximum exposure even for an electrical worker (the public's exposure level is 10-fold lower) is 1.0 mW/cm2 for no more than 6 minutes. This is equivalent to 10 W/m2. In my opinion even this is an extremely high exposure, which is the reason that the maximum time to be in this very high level is limited to 6 minutes."

So, it is all a big mystery. I can surmise that it had to do with national defense, but whether it was incoming missile defense or for the newly opened National Security Agency's data-mining program, we do not know; and anyway, I do not have the tools it would take to expose the perpetrators. Knowing who the perpetrators are would not undo the damage to our health, so it is a nonissue. Too much time has gone by. It may sound melodramatic, but over time I became tired of being afraid. By hearing about the threats that had been leveled against some of those involved in researching our EMF radiation poisoning, I had been living in fear of powers that might not like me agitating, or that I had witnessed public endangerment. I did not know definitively what we had or had not seen or been witnesses to, but obviously details were being kept hidden. Were company actions sanctioned or were they not? Why were the powers that be not forthcoming with information or help? As much as we liked the fun and adventure of Europe, California seemed like a good place to meld into a sea of normalcy. I had a feeling we were running away and looking back over our shoulders. I was sure this would not be the last we'd hear about our radiation poisoning event.

The government had to know that using radiation emissions at highly dangerous levels would have repercussions somewhere. The damage was not suffered by those who made the decisions, so it just doesn't matter. I suppose I have to leave the "Why did this happen?" a mystery.

A couple of facts I found interesting: The mast is still on the barn, and to date, does not have an owner label on it, although all other masts in the area are labeled.

President Bush promoted a new Protect America bill passed in March of 2007 that funded a new surveillance program, Prism. Does this new program have anything to do with the *experiments* I felt?

While compiling this report, we came across a letter, written in 2005 by a physician in Bamberg, to the German Prime Minister. This letter, supported by 185 local German physicians, highlights a crisis situation in patient health associated with EMF in Oberfranken. We lived twenty-six miles from the physician who wrote the letter. We lived in Oberfranken. Is this the smoking gun? This letter was written less than a year prior to our moving to the region. This is the *stew* we moved into.

Date: 10.07.2005
An open letter to Edmund Stoiber

To Prime Minister Dr. Edmund Stoiber
State Chancellery
P.O.. Box 220011
80535 Munich

A most urgent evaluation of severe health damage caused by pulsed high frequency electromagnetic fields (Mobile telephone base stations, DECT telephones, W-LAN, Bluetooth etc.) far beneath the recommended limit values.

Dear Mr. Prime Minister

Please allow me to address you personally in the name of many physicians.

For eight months physicians in Oberfranken and other places have made extremely worrying observations on patients who live in the periphery of mobile phone base stations. After the initial evaluations at locations in Forchheim, Hirschaid, Walsdorf, Memmelsdorf and Bamberg questions and tests were carried out on 356 residents living under long term exposure in their homes or at work, living in over 40 locations in the whole of Oberfranken

Meanwhile some 64 doctors and physicians in Hofer, 30 in Lichtenfelser, 61 in Coburger, 20 Natives of Bayreuth and country-wide have supported the Bamberger appeal. The results of all these medical evaluations are as follows:

Many humans get sick from emissions far below the recommended limit values, which consider only thermal effects, and we have a sickness picture with characteristic symptom combinations, which are new to us physicians,.

People suffer from one, several or many of the following symptoms:

Sleep disturbances, tiredness, concentration impairment, forgetfulness, problem with finding words, depressive tendencies, tinnitus, sudden loss of hearing, hearing loss, giddiness, nose bleeds, visual disturbances, frequent infections, sinusitis, joint and limb pains, nerve and soft

tissue pains, feeling of numbness, heart rhythm disturbances, increased blood pressure, hormonal disturbances, night-time sweat, nausea.

The following statements strengthened the suspicion:

Frequently many resident got sick at the same time with these symptoms (f.ins. in Schweinfurt: Eselhöhe, in Kulmbach: Senior housing estate Mainpark, in Hof: Köesseinestrasse, in Forchheim: Orstei Burk).
Many patients reported prompt, improvement immediately the exposures ceases (temporary moving away from home, removal of Dect telephones, using shielding, permanently moving away).

After moving away from the exposure, physicians were able to prove, by re-testing the patients, the normalization of blood pressure, heart rhythm, hormone disturbances, visual disturbances, neurological symptoms, blood picture, among other things

Many family physicians have removed, in the course of the last months, their patients DECT telephones and have found that people afterwards were free from headache, concentration impairment, forgetfulness, unrest, Tinnitus, sleep disturbances, etc.

Thereafter we directly asked for investigations to be arranged at the locations, by the responsible authorities (Federal Office for radiation protection, Federal Ministry for environment, nature protection and reactor safety, members of the radiation protection commission and the WHO).
Despite the serious, medical suspicion all the authorities refused to investigate the z. T. intolerable life situation of the residents locally.

Official health investigations have **NOT** been carried out at one single mobile base station location in Germany! The SSK and the BfS have thus no knowledge of the effects of the long-term-exposure on the residents. From medical view is this unacceptable.

I therefore turn to you with the request for assistance for our desperate patients.
We, physicians in Oberfranken, are ready to help.

Please will you arrange, that investigations of the state of health of the residents at some locations in Bavaria will be carried out immediately.
This is not a question of some "unfortunate individual cases", but a medical disaster spreading in all parts of the population!

For the investigation of our suspicion it must also be possible to switch off individual transmitters. From a medical view an emergency situation is present, which requires rapid action by all political forces.

I ask you please, to immediately set in motion the necessary steps, and thereby minimizing health damage to many children, young people and adults.
Faithfully
Dr. Cornelia Waldmann-Selsam
Karl-May-Str.48   96049 Bamberg

Anne Mills

Back Home to California

As much as we enjoyed living in Europe, every weekend in a different country or at a different festival, we were glad to get back to our friends and family. It was so wonderful to be, once again, in close proximity to our only son and his new wife. It was wonderful to be by our parents as they aged. We had fulfilled the contract for Eric's employment, and I was looking to find a job of my own. I was also hoping for a return to what I thought of as *normal*. But quickly I began to see that *any* experience changes forever our perspective, and that perspective, in turn, colors new experiences. There is no *new normal*, only new experiences. Our perspective, now based on our time living in another country, along with our new health concerns, would forever change how we moved forward. The one foreseen normal was much better weather. Conversely, and almost weirdly, I realized how much I missed cobblestones beneath my boots.

Eric was back working at the local Siemens office to finish out his four-year contract. We found a new rental home in Walnut Creek. Our thinking was that California would have less EMF radiation, but that proved not to be true. Right away, the humming heard every night still kept sleep at bay. So, to help alleviate the problem, we bought a White Noise machine. With this little machine I tried to mask the EMF humming with sounds like traffic, or a flowing brook, (which made me have to go to the bathroom). My favorite was the sound of rain. It did help some. What would help more is not have the humming. I was not getting the intense symptoms and pains I had experienced in Germany, but not being able to sleep was nonetheless a danger to my body, as without sleep I cannot produce Melatonin. Not having Melatonin impedes the body from being able to rejuvenate and fight off illness. We were living in Walnut Creek, and like everyone else, we had to grocery shop. In the parking lot of the little strip mall by our new home, we found ourselves staring at a metal cell tower. It's about three times the circumference of a telephone pole, only about as tall as a two-story building, short for a mast, and disguised as a flag pole. On one side of this cell tower was placed a 5" x 8" label warning not to stand close. This radiating cell tower was among the little bistro tables and chairs of a well-known coffee house. We were shocked. We did not shop there anymore. (We later found that the radiation from that short cell tower maxed out our radiation meter.)

I was now faced with radiation too high to comfortably sleep, and reluctantly acknowledged that I needed a Faraday cage. I did not want to go back into a cage. We decided to try a fabric shelter. Unlike the Faraday cages Eric built, a fabric shelter would be soft and flowing and maybe not seem so cage-like. We purchased a fabric shelter from LESSEMF.com. This seemed to help some at first, and it may be a good shelter for some, but with my sensitivities, I needed something more protective. It was at this time that we researched and purchased our first EMF radiation meter. We were only living there a couple of months when we found that our new neighborhood was in a fight against a cell tower company. This cell tower (*masts* as I had known them in Germany) was to be installed in front of the Catholic Church only a block away from our new home. I believe that we were all lucky in finding this information, as the church was going to have it installed without much notification to people in the neighborhood.

I lent my time, knowledge, and research material on the health dangers of EMF to the small coalition of locals fighting this tower. We believed everyone in the area had a right to know what was coming into their midst, and made up fliers and went door to door in several neighborhoods. We wrote newspaper articles to inform the public. Sadly, the cell tower went in despite all our efforts. Once again too many close cell towers, too much man-made pulsed microwave radiation, became a health issue and we decided we needed to move. Our neighborhood was all EMF'd up.

So how is it that the wireless industry is allowed to pollute the environment without the approval of citizens in local neighborhoods? The Communication Act of 1996. This act nullified nearly all local input for decision-making by corporations and the Federal Communications Commission, even when there might be adverse health effects brought on by their practices and installations. This is why you see cell towers camouflaged as trees. Aesthetics is about the only viable justification locals can use to fight against cell phone towers. Citizens are not allowed to argue on the bases of health risks. As of the date of this writing, the wireless industry is attempting to push through legislation in all the state houses throughout the nation eliminating restrictions on cell tower and micro-cell installations, to enable 5G. The highest levels of political contributions are not from *Big Pharma* or *Big Oil* or *Big Agra*, but rather from the wireless industry. The FCC has been a captured agency for decades. So, there is no agency protecting us. At least in Germany there was an agency that monitored radiation levels, where in the US there is no policing whatsoever. The industry is left to monitor itself—or not.

Moving Again

We decided to rent in a more remote and quieter area to get away from high EMF radiation. We packed and moved for the fourth time in five years. Sadly, I was getting good at this. About this time, Eric lost his job at Siemens. He had only been back in the States six months, so Siemens determined that this was not long enough for him to have earned a severance.

Though in the middle of Walnut Creek, the little studio we found was on a large piece of property with a creek running through it and many large oak trees. There were no close neighbors, so we were not concerned about neighbor EMF radiation. In our move, we took the fabric shelter and hoped it would work in the new home, but we were sadly disappointed. This fabric shelter would be good for traveling, so we kept it. Eric decided that for our new house he would build another Faraday cage. Learning from his mistakes with earlier cage-building attempts in Germany, Eric built a Faraday cage in our Walnut Creek home that was spacious, solid, and very effective.

Based on our experience to date, we were mainly focused on radiation from cell towers. But we had learned that it wasn't just cell tower masts to look out for, but cell phones as well, and radiation from neighborhood Wi-Fi networks and smart meters. We thought we had information on the closest cell towers, but I was still feeling EMF. Sadly, and unluckily, the move to the new house coincided with the rollout of smart meters to that neighborhood. To our advantage, our smart meter was on an outbuilding a couple of car lengths from our studio. Even so, it was still spewing radiation into the yard where I might have otherwise spent time.

So, I joined the local fight against smart meters. Eric and I had the pleasure of meeting and working with some wonderful people. As I was not as sensitive then as I am now, I was able to go to a court hearing against smart meters with Ellie Marks and Lloyd Morgan, new colleagues in the fight against EMF. My actual time in the courtroom had to be significantly limited due to the high radiation there. This outing left me ill for a couple of days, recuperating in the cage.

I was able to grocery shop as long as I did so early in the morning when there were fewer shoppers with cell phones. Even though I took this precaution, I needed to spend time in the cage once I returned home. I found that I was spending more and more time in the Faraday cage, sometimes up to twenty hours a day. It turns out that California EMF levels during the day were much higher than those in Europe. People here have their faces in a cell phones more often than people in Europe. I could not escape microwave radiation and I was feeling ill a good part of each day. I found myself going into the cage to get away from the constant buzzing. But spending a good deal of time in a Faraday cage is depressing.

Noticing my depression, Eric took a day off work to search for an area where we could live that did not have cell reception. We drove for hours, every so often stopping to check radiation levels. To this end, we found ourselves moving again, to a very rural area, this one three plus hours away from the Bay Area. *Knock on wood*, this area had been ignored, to large extent, by industry.

We moved to our new home in early 2011, our fifth move in five years. Yikes. We now owned a home in a forest. The biggest change and challenge in this move was that Eric and I would not be living together. Eric had a new job in Emeryville, and the three-hour drive between work and home rendered a daily commute impossible. We found a small apartment in Alameda for Eric. He drove home on Thursday, than back to the Bay Area on Monday at 6:00 AM, rain or shine on his motorcycle. This was the first time we lived apart in our thirty-plus years of marriage.

Almost ironically, we were not in our new, rural home for a month before the smart meter began making its debut. Eric and I spoke with our new neighbors, being frank about why we were asking them to opt out of smart meters. If they got a smart meter, it would put me back in the cage. We were quite lucky: our wonderful neighbors, all three of them, opted out for us. We felt blessed.

Breast Cancer

In early 2012 I discovered I had breast cancer. I also had a simultaneous complication of a persistent and painful stomach problem that had surfaced the previous Christmas. Because we lived so far out, I had to drive myself to tests two-plus hours away. We worried about this forewarned cancer, and my persistent stomach pain. Even with all the tests being taken, the doctors had no idea what caused my stomach issue. The doctors thought I might have a tumor close by my uterus.

It was very frightening for me to know I had *The Big C*, but I was nearly as frightened by the MRIs I needed to verify my diagnosis. The high EMF radiation from the tests at the doctor's office made me ill. Though it seems I was not then as sensitive to EMF as I am now, I still became ill when visiting the doctor. I would wait outside in our car, asking the nurse to come get me when they were ready for me. I had to explain my sensitivity and hope for understanding. They finally determined that I needed to have surgery to repair the stomach-tumor issue prior to having a mastectomy for the breast cancer. It turns out that although there were no known cases of cancer in my family, the tests showed I had breast cancer. The doctors wanted me to have chemo and radiation. I gave the doctors an emphatic "no" on the radiation, but not feeling I had a choice, I issued a nod to chemotherapy.

Before my surgery, Eric went to the hospitals and spoke with the nursing staff. He informed them of my sensitivities. Sutter hospital, at both sites, took measures to ensure that I had as little exposure to EMFs as possible. For overnight stays they put me in rooms away from the break room, which housed a microwave for staff. They put a sign on the door asking those entering to turn off their cell phones. In the one instance when I shared a room, they told the other patient and their guests that I could not tolerate cell phones or wireless devices. In the instance when they did not have a room without EMF, they gave me my own room in the ICU area. The doctors and nurses were wonderful and we were grateful.

During the surgery for my stomach tumor, doctors found that it was not a tumor at all, but rather that my appendix had burst sometime around Christmas. I was still alive because my colon had wrapped around the appendix and contained the burst. This was a miracle. Ten days after this first surgery, I had another, a mastectomy. I totally blame the cancer on the poisoning event in Germany. Throughout convalescence, Eric would come home each weekend and cook, clean, and do laundry. He would take me for rides and make me food for the coming week. I think he loves me.

Disability

It turns out that I could no longer work due to my EHS Radiation sickness. In 2010 we decided that I would apply for disability. With the help of my physician in Germany, Dr. Horst Eger; my wonderful lawyer; and my brave husband; I was granted disability benefits based on Electromagnetic HyperSensitivity in 2012. It took two years of work and an appeal. It was believed that I was the first in the United States, maybe in the world, to be granted permanent EHS disability. We were cautioned not to speak of it to anyone. (See chapter on Disability)

Rural Area gets All EMF*d Up

When we first moved to this rural area, I was able to do all my own shopping. I was able to go to the post office for stamps and send packages. I used to get gas for my car, and drive around town doing chores. I was an active member of the local gym, taking Pilates classes. I met girlfriends at the local café or restaurant for brunch or a basil martini. I enjoyed taking art classes and being a participant in the local festivals. Eric and I could attend concerts at the wonderful local theatre.

As well, Eric and I volunteered to be on the local trail clean-up crew. Our area is host to many shops that sell art and I loved to peruse their offerings. I walked our German Shepherd on the streets of our rural community. Eric and I supported local restaurants. I was a car show judge at three consecutive annual auto shows. I was a board member and secretary for the local Community Center. That was all so fun for me.

Unfortunately, our area now has Wi-Fi antennas attached to many local buildings. Thus, I can no longer do any of the above listed activities, as the EMF radiation is too high for my sensitivities. The area is all EMF'd up. I can no longer be an active social member of our community. I am dependent on my husband, Eric, to do all our shopping and run errands. I can no longer drive my car through town; I can only be out in our van with EMF-shielded windows. Once again, I am cloistered.

Where Do We Go?

Until now, we have been lucky to have lived in this rurally situated house, relatively safe from EMF for eight years. A few months ago I started experiencing symptoms at night: hot flashes, headaches, teeth ache, insomnia, tinnitus. Our EMF meters indicated that there was no RF present and that we were safe. Was my health failing or was this RF that the meter couldn't read? I started writing all ill feelings in a diary, which showed it happened on a timed and scheduled basis. Eric purchased a new meter that showed a wider range of frequencies. Until the new meter arrived, we found ourselves sleeping in our vehicle on a friend's remote property. When the new meter arrived it showed that we were in fact being exposed to high levels of EMF. This proved that my ill feelings were environmental. Until we found the source of this new radiation, we had to shield the house. Eric applied aluminum screen on windows and doors on the side of the house facing the direction the meter was indicating. He also lined our faraday cage with a layer of aluminum screen over the existing hardware cloth. Once again, we could sleep at home. We are now investigating exactly where the source of this emission is coming from.

We just found out that a cell tower is going to be erected on a hill four miles away. The world's three largest wireless providers will affix their antennae to this tower. We are facing very real EMF dangers once again. What do we do? Do Eric and I spend the money and try to protect our home? What if the money we spend is not enough to ensure protection? After spending the money to protect ourselves, can we afford to move? If we move, where do we go? We do not believe many will fight the cell tower, as not many know about the dangers of invisible radiation. Will there be locals who voice concern? I wrote letters to our local newspaper and posted fliers against smart meters. How many people paid attention? A small town can be a difficult place to voice minority opinion. If they don't put the cell tower there in town, will they propose to have it closer to our home? Once again we are fighting windmills of big money. We are scared and tired of continually looking over our shoulder for the next big threat of EMF. When will *The People* have a say about what is built in the local environment?

Technology isn't bad—the issue is how we decide to use it, overuse it, or abuse it. The issue is about how it harms us. Only when everyone is aware of the health dangers that cell towers and wireless devices pose, will we be able to stand united and fight Big Money and its forced irradiation. Soon we might all be staring at a 5G mini tower in our front yard. It's our health and lifestyle versus corporate greed. We must become aware, acknowledge and do our part, share knowledge, and take a stand for ourselves and those we care about.

So YaY!, I wrote the story I needed to get outside of myself. I can hold it in my hand instead of in my head. I want to thank you, my reader, for allowing me to share this true story. Getting the experience outside of myself has helped. I feel more open.

Thank you for sharing in this journey. As I could find no reason for this poisoning event, I hope others can use some part of my painful experience to make a better life for themselves and others. That is why, I believe, it happened to me. I am hoping that by getting this information outside of me I can turn toward sharing the magic and light that Eric and I experienced while living in Europe. Now, finally, I can write the other book I want to write, a fun adventure about a loving couple. I think I will call the next sharing, "A Cheery Bowl of Hamlets".

> Though I can offer no rosy outlook
> My hope is that my terrible experience
> Will give others insight, foreknowledge,
> And an impetus to protect themselves.
>
> My hope is that those whose lives have already
> Been negatively impacted by industry,
> know they are not alone.
>
> My hope is that someone in a position
> to regulate our precarious polluted system
> Finds the consciousness and strength to do so.
>
> …and that those who knew the dangers
> and gave their consent to experimenting on humanity
> —I will be your thorn
>
> Anne.

Part 2

What is ElectroMagnetic Hyper Sensitivity (EHS)

Because I was diagnosed in Europe, I have always referred to my illness as Electromagnetic HyperSensitivity (EHS), as this is how it was introduced to me. The U.S. Government refers to the illness as EMS or Electromagnetic Sensitivity. EHS is also known as "Radio Wave Sickness" and "Microwave Sickness." As many of the symptoms of EHS are the same ones experienced as we age, Dr. Magda Havas calls it "Rapid Aging Syndrome," or RAS. EHS has a wide range of symptoms and every person experiences it differently. EHS was officially identified in the 1970s by Russian doctors to describe an occupational malady experienced by workers who were exposed to microwave or radiofrequency radiation.

With EHS, the body exhibits negative health symptoms when subjected to electrical and/or man made pulsed non-ionized radiation (EMF). EMF emissions are broadcast into our environment by cell phone towers, wireless devices and appliances. Electromagnetic Field (EMF) radiation, like other environmental pollutants, poisons our body and all living things. EMF radiation is invisible, and it bounces and reflects off surfaces the same way that light does. You can't see or smell EMF radiation, and most people can't hear or feel it.

EMF radiation is also quite ignored in our society at this writing, as it is something that the telecom industry has done a great job of hiding, and the media and politicians go along with their crime. Most U.S. physicians have not been trained in EHS, its causes, or symptoms. All physicians we were in contact with in Germany, from the general practitioner to specialty physicians, were aware of EMF negative health impacts. Unlike Europe, the research done in the U.S. on Electromagnetic

Sensitivity is largely paid for by industry and is biased in their favor. The World Health Organization (WHO) estimates that 3% of the world's population sufferers from EHS. Per the WHO, in population-based surveys, the prevalence of EHS has ranged from 1.5% in Sweden to 13.3% in Taiwan. Per the U.S. National Institute of Health, EHS is closely connected to another illness called Multiple Chemical Sensitivity (MCS), a toxic-immune syndrome caused by exposure to chemical agents: https://www.ncbi.nlm.nih.gov/pubmed/26372109

"Our data clearly shows that EHS and MCS should be recognized as genuine somatic pathological entities; that patients with EHS and/or MCS are nonpsychosomatic nor psychiatric patients; and probably that EHS and MCS are two etiopathogenic aspects of a single pathological disorder." www.ehs-mcs.org/fichiers/1454070991_Reliable_biomarkers.pdf

What in my environment causes EHS:

Though I was initially poisoned by local cell towers, the exposure left me sensitive to all things wireless. This includes radiating devices, such as a cell phones, routers, and cordless phones. Wireless devices are synonymous to radiation; they do not work without emitting radiation. All along the freeways, cell phone tower masts spew high levels of radiation. Every store you enter has credit card machines, door sensors, security, phones, hand-held inventory management, and wireless computers. Did you know that most supermarket lottery machines and ATM machines are wireless? Most vehicles now have wireless computer systems, tracking, area sensors and Blue Tooth. This will only get worse as vehicles become autonomous. Some EHS sufferers are also sensitive to electrical appliances and lights, which do emit ELF (dirty electricity). So, basically, wireless radiation, which can cause EHS, is nearly impossible to escape.

Becoming EHS sensitive is not brought on by natural sun and earth ionizing radiation. The background radiation given off from natural means is so small our radiation meters can't pick it up. We are specifically speaking man made pulsed non-ionizing radiation.

Why does EHS occur?

The body, being made of water and electrical in nature, has not evolved to put up with a constant bath of the new man-made sources of radiation. I have been told that EMF radiation is cumulative in the body, and it does not naturally slough off. EMF's bring down the body's immune system, so when your body is depleted of the ability to ward off and heal itself, when your body cannot deal with as much radiation as it's subjected to, you start feeling ill. It is obvious that more research needs to be done. The fact that a large percent of EHS sufferers are women is thought to be due to biological or chromosomal differences.

Eric and I did not associate our feeling ill with anything we had done with a wireless device. Most people don't do a timeline as to when they started feeling ill, so it is difficult to come to the causation. They are unable to say "Oh, I started feeling ill when I got the new phone,'' or "I started getting ill after the smart meter was put on my bedroom wall." Most people don't put the two together—radiation and feeling ill. As EHS is not a well-known malady, and most physicians are not trained in environmental medicine, they don't look for an environmental cause for symptoms. Instead of suggesting the patient take the cordless phone off the head of the bed, they might be given a pill for the insomnia or cream for their eczema.

To be more proactive in your own health, it makes sense to note if your heart palpitations started when you got a new wireless router for your laptop. Did your headaches or vertigo start when purchased a new car with WiFi hot spot? Our American doctors need to be trained in how environmental pollutants adversely impact our health. This includes electromagnetic field radiation as well as multiple chemicals. In 2006, the World Health Organization reported "estimates that more than 13 million deaths annually are due to preventable environmental causes. Nearly one third of death and disease in the least developed regions is due to environmental causes." It would be welcomed if a doctor would try to discover if there was an environmental trigger for symptoms. If you have an open-minded doctor, give them all the information you can find on EMF and its health effects. If your physician is not open-minded, search for one who is. Be proactive in your own health. There are many peer-reviewed scientific/medical research papers you could share with your physician at www.EHTrust.org, or www.MDSafeTech.org.

In 2011, the World Health Organization (WHO) classified EMF radiation as a possible 2B carcinogen. Now, in 2019, scientists have compiled research documents that point to EMF radiation being a Class 1 Human carcinogen. "When considered with recent animal experimental evidence, the recent epidemiological studies strengthen and support the conclusion that RFR should be categorized as carcinogenic to humans (IARC Class1)." www.saferemr.com/2018/04/recent-research

Symptoms

Symptoms of EHS are many, and some are synonymous with MS, MCS, Lyme disease or even the flu. You might experience one or several of the following symptoms, maybe for the brief time you are exposed or sometimes hours or days after exposure:

- insomnia
- tinnitis – your ears ring to a point of distraction, sometimes many different pitches
- headaches – whole head, just spikes, or sometimes just where you held your phone.
- head pressure–A heavy headed strong pressure or squeeze feeling.
- fog head–A numb minded, swimmy headed feeling that leaves one unfocused
- nausea
- hot flashes
- extreme fatigue
- body aches and pains
- heart palpitations and arrhythmias
- tunnel vision and eye problems
- difficulty concentrating
- memory loss
- nose bleeds
- allergy/asthma
- night sweats
- confusion / depression / anxiety triggering fight or flight
- hair loss – overall thinning
- skin rashes or unusual redness, itching or swelling – eczema
- overall degradation of immune system

EMF exposure has been linked to autism, ADHD, epilepsy, diabetes, cancers, thyroid problems, neurological disorders, multiple sclerosis, heart irregularities, Alzheimers, Parkinsons, miscarriages, cardiovascular issues, fertility issues, photosensitivity, MCS, and food allergies.
www.emfanalysis.com/EHS-symptoms

It has been known since the 1970s that exposure to even very low levels of EMF can cause a breakdown in the Blood Brain Barrier allowing toxins that would normally be screened out, to enter the brain.
www.rfsafe.com/cell-phone-radiation-damages-blood-brain-barrier/

Voltage-Gated Calcium Channels
"Now [I have found] 26 [papers]" "They all show that EMFs work by activating what are called voltage-gated calcium channels (VGCCs). These are channels in the outer membrane of the cell, the plasma membrane that surrounds all our cells. When they're activated, they open up and allow calcium to flow into the cell. It's the excess calcium in the cell which is responsible for most if not all of the [biological effects]." Dr. Martin Pall.

The highest density of VGCCs is in our nervous system and that is also the system most sensitive to EMF. When the VGCCs are activated in the brain, they produce effects such as anxiety, depression, and links to autism and Alzheimer. Our heart is another organ that has high density in VGCCs. If you find you are experiencing any unusual heart palps, cardiac arrhythmias, atrial fibrillation, fast or slow heartbeat, you need to take immediate steps to lower your exposure to EMFs and see a doctor. Another area of VGCCs is the reproductive organs, particularly in males, and it has been shown to impair or reduces fertility. You can read all of Dr. Martin Pall's findings by doing a search for "Dr. Martin Pall." His papers can be found on all reputable EMF sites like www.emfsafetynetwork.org or www.ehtrust.org.

I believe that EMFs need to be looked at closely by the medical institutions regarding the growing number of the younger populace experiencing heart issues. Stated in The ARIC Community Surveillance Study, "Younger patients, ranging in age from 35 to 54 years of age, accounted for 27 percent of all people hospitalized with heart attacks in the U.S. between 1995-1999, and increased to 32 percent between 2010-2014, with a greater increase among women compared to men. During the study period, heart attack incidence for women rose from 21 percent to 31 percent; for men, the incidence increased from 30 percent to 33 percent." (found in the Twenty Year Trends and Sex Differences in Young Adults Hospitalized with Acute Myocardial Infarction - www.ahajournals.org/doi/10.1161/CIRCULATIONAHA.118.037137)

Unusual Symptoms of EHS
Loss of Motor Skills, Vocabulary, and Sense of Smell

Several symptoms of EHS can be mistakenly interpreted as flu or pneumonia, when in fact they could have been brought on by exposure to EMF. If the medicine my physician gives me is not working, I would also consider removing the wireless devices from my bedroom. As a matter of habit, I turn off most electrical breakers to the house to cut down on the dirty electricity.

Because the symptoms of EHS are synonymous with many other ailments, a physician might prescribe something to help one of the symptoms and not see the overall picture. You might have started off with only one or two symptoms, as I did. They sneak up on you and don't seem so bad taken one at a time, until you realize that you were fine just a couple months ago but now you feel quite ill.

Vertigo. At the end of 2006 and into 2007, when first experiencing the cell tower poisoning, I found that upon waking I had terrible balance. Everything felt swimmy and my feet were difficult to keep under my body. As this was one of my first symptoms, I did not give it much credit. Now I only feel vertigo and head pressure when entering a store or office building that has high EMF, but not always. I recently came upon research papers that not only brought vertigo to mind, but explained why I had this experience. Dr. Belpomme's study (p.260) says that diminished blood flow to the brain (hypoperfusion) is a biomarker for EHS.
www.ehs-mcs.org/fichiers/1454070991-Reliable_biomarkers.pdf

A couple years ago I found myself at a local community gathering of about forty people. Eric and I had attended many of their dinners and the group was always so nice in accommodating my EHS issue. This evening I was by myself. Even though I asked nicely for others to turn their phones off, not everyone thinks this is an issue. Unknown to me, someone at dinner refused to turn their phone off. I didn't feel the normal warning of heavy symptoms, but subtle spiky headache sensations. When it was time to leave, I felt inebriated though I had not had alcohol. I felt vertigo and blurry vision. It took me over half an hour, sitting alone in the car, to feel that I had recovered my senses enough to drive home.

Loss of sense of smell. I lost my sense of smell starting with the poisoning event in 2007. It was only later that I learned that this, too, is another symptom of the EMF poisoning. On one hand, it didn't bother me that I couldn't smell offensive odors such as when the farmers sprayed their fields with manure but not being able to smell food was upsetting. Without aroma, food was not as appealing. I didn't get the real tang of cheese or the essence of a ripe tomato. I would walk into a bakery and get nothing; no fresh baked bread or scent of cinnamon. Smells bring back memories and now not having that ability was depressing. I was without the ability to smell for about two years, and only after I minimized EMF exposure and started healing did my sense of smell return. The first thing I did smell was skunk, and nothing reeked as sweet as realizing that my nose was back. Of course, cry when you lose it; cry when you get it back.

<u>Loss of vocabulary</u>. After the initial poisoning, one of my main symptoms was loss of vocabulary. I found myself without the ability to express myself as I had lost all known words. Small words, such as "there" or "hungry" or "hurt" were gone. I took up extensive reading in an effort to relearn my vocabulary. Even though it is years after the poisoning event, in areas where the EMF is intense, I have had experienced loss of vocabulary. People ask me a question, and I *know* they expect an answer in return, but have no idea what they said. I find myself without the ability to string thoughts into a sentence and vocalize. When this happens, I feel not only brain fog and am numb minded, but feel anxious and overwhelmed.

<u>Fight or flight</u>. I learned that fight or flight is another symptom of EHS, can occur instantly, and can be taken by others as rude. It is a symptom that comes on fast, gives no warning. In this mode, I either run from a confusing situation or am confrontational in scary situations. (see chapter on "Fight or Flight and Depression")

<u>Loss of motor skills</u>. There have been a few instances when the EMFs were so high I would lose the ability to control my body; I have just fallen, like a rag doll, to the ground. I am aware of what is happening, I know that people are talking, and sometimes understand words, but I can only answer in short sentences, like "get me out." Even saying "get me out" takes a lot of effort to put thought to words. It is scary to not have control of one's self, have to depend on others to take care of you, when a minute ago you were normal. Luckily, I was with co-workers and friends, and they knew what to do. They took me outside to a safe area away from EMFs and in about half an hour I recovered. It turns out that someone we did not know walked

into our work space with a cell phone that put out huge EMF. He EMF'd the whole place and as a result, I collapsed.

This should demonstrate that as much as you might like to keep this illness a secret, you might want to consider having someone close at hand that is aware of your health situation; someone that can help if some unforeseen medical symptom arises. In point, from then on, I carried my radiation meter that has a sound function. If I had had the meter, I would have been forewarned and been able to leave the area, i.e., protect myself. This same loss of motor skills and vocabulary happened once in a sandwich shop and another while in line at a store. Eric had to assist me out of the area and it took about two hours to be back to a semblance of normal.

<u>Hearing EMF Frequencies</u>. I can hear EMF frequencies. I had no idea what the different hums were that I was experiencing but it drove me crazy trying to find the source. Different frequencies have different pitches, as I explained in the first half of the book, My Journey. I don't know how common this is or how it works but in my investigation have found that Allan Frey, from Cornell University studied the issue for twenty years. In 1962 he wrote:
"The "hearing" of electromagnetic waves is an established fact. It appears that this takes place by direct stimulation of the nervous system, perhaps in the brain, thus bypassing the ear and much of the associated hearing system."
(To find, Search: Human Auditory System Response to Modulated Electromagnetic Energy Allan Frey pdf 1962)

<u>Suicide</u>: One of the symptoms of EHS is depression. Suicide rates have risen exponentially, and I am sure there could be quite a few reasons for the numbers. I would hate to think that any of those deaths can be contributed to electromagnetic radiation, an environmental pollutant that can be controlled and protected against.

Mr Trower, a scientific adviser to the Radiation Research Trust, said he is convinced the (suicide) deaths are related to an illness caused by the waves after investigating five suicide "clusters" across the UK and Ireland. "I am 99 per cent sure," said Mr Trower, who contributed to the BBC Panorama program WiFi: A Warning Signal. "I think I can link them all together and I think it's a viable reason to look into. We know the suicide rates are rising. The increase in suicides does match the speed of low level microwaves. It's happening in every country in the world, not just Bridgend." He has investigated links between 182 suicides and electrosensitivity, a condition thought to affect three per cent of the population....
www.eon3emfblog.net/smeter-moratorium-laws-spread-emfs-suicides-digest-for-3-4-11

Per the Washington Post, "Nearly 45,000 suicides occurred in the United States in 2016. That is more than twice the number of homicides, making it the 10th-leading cause of death. Among people ages 15 to 34, suicide is the second-leading cause of death. In more than half of all deaths in 27 states, the people had no known mental health condition when they ended their lives. In half of the states, suicide among people age 10 and older increased more than 30 percent."

According to a study in 2010, five to eight times as many high school and college students meet the criteria for diagnosis of major depression and/or anxiety disorder compared to 50 years ago. This increased psychopathology is not the result of changed diagnostic criteria.
www.psychologytoday.com/us/blog/freedom-learn/201001/the-decline-play-and-rise-in-childrens-mental-disorders. (Angela Tsiang)

<u>Acute EHS</u> A wonderful website, EHSIdaho.com states: "…symptoms as multiple sensory up-regulation, which is very common in <u>acute cases of EHS</u>. The most common conditions of sensory up-regulation are:

1. Photophobia and/or Scotopic sensitivity syndrome (visual sensitivity)
2. Hyperacusis (heightened sense of hearing)
3. Hyperosmia (heightened sense of smell)
4. Hypergeusia (heightened sense of taste)
5. Hyperesthesia/Photosensitivity (heightened skin sensitivity)
6. Multiple Chemical Sensitivity (extreme sensitivity to chemicals)
7. Vibroacoustic Disease (VAD) (systemic pathology from low frequency noise)

Just as not everyone experiences EHS the same, not everyone's EMF poisoning event is the same. I have met people that have EHS due to multiple smart meters being placed on their homes. I have met people that suffer from EHS due to a workplace environment overload of radiation. Many that suffer from EHS find that they were left susceptible due to a head injury, concussion, or from the heavy metal residue left in the body from medical procedures. I have now met several people that became sensitive from exposure to radiation in a hospital environment coupled with their own cell phone use. Other than abstinence of EMF, I have not heard of or know of an instance where once you have become hypersensitive you can heal and not feel ill effects from EMF. I believe that if you stay away from EMFs, the symptoms disappear, but when re-exposure happens, you are liable to have your symptoms reappear; at least that is what happens to me. I feel fine until I am around EMFs, then I feel ill.

I don't know why the symptoms are not always the same, but I can only surmise that it is due to the radiation frequency, radiation energy levels, and a body's particular weaknesses. Some EMF exposures make every tooth in my mouth hurt. Sometimes the symptom is a feeling of pressure in the chest area. Occasionally EMF exposure causes every bone in my body to hurt, or my shoulders to ache. So I guess that these symptoms that mark us as having EHS, radiation sickness, is what my doctor referred to as being "the canary in the coal mine." Some feel the invisible EMF monster in the room; the phantom that others can't detect. If you are one that can't feel the EMF radiation, but feel the after-effects, please purchase and carry an EMF radiation meter. It can save you untold hours of discomfort. One doctor told me that EMFs are adversely affecting everyone in the same way whether you can feel it or not. I interpret my symptoms as my body finding a way to tell me that the area is not safe; I need to get out. I curse my symptoms as they keep me from living fully; I thank my symptoms for the warning.

Learn all you can about your sensitivities and share your knowledge with those you want to spend time with, so you can socialize safely. Talk with other EHS survivors to get more ideas on what might also work for you. (see the More Information chapter)

It is a most difficult thing to open up and admit that you have sensitivity to something that one can not see or smell, is not generally accepted, and is difficult to diagnose. Holding a secret like this is painful. Know that you are a normal person whose body has an exaggerated response to the pollutant EMF. I believe EHS is a malady where most who have it *do not know*, those that do know *are afraid to say*, and those that do not have it *don't usually believe*.

Please know you are not alone. You are a survivor.
To read other EHS survivor stories or to let others know your story, go to: www.Mast-Victims.org.

How to Protect Your Home and Work Environment

As my EMF radiation poisoning event took place in Europe, I was fortunate to be under the care of doctors knowledgeable in Electromagnetic Sensitivity. We were told by Dr. Heinlein, Chief Physician at the University of Wuerzberg, Klinikum in Coberg, Germany, that "there is not a lot we can do to stop from being bombarded by EMFs emitted by external antenna and cell phone masts. What you *do* have control over, is your home. The best and fastest way to help yourself is to ensure that you are not polluting your own home space." The illness and subsequent protection of self might feel overwhelming at first, but once you take action, you will start feeling better. When you start feeling better, you will remember your normal self and even realize that many discomforts you lived with were associated with EMF.

Awareness, Acknowledgement, Avoidance of EMF

Acknowledgement of the dangers of Electromagnetic Field radiation is a big step in protection efforts. Man-made pulsed microwave radiation is not natural, and our bodies have not evolved to live with them. Electromagnetic Hypersensitivity, or Microwave Sickness (EHS) points to the fact that some people feel the effects of EMF and some do not. Second is the **awareness** of where the EMF is being emitted. We as a society find ourselves increasingly dependent on wireless devices and due to this, EMF's are rather difficult to get away from. Cell phones and cordless phones, baby monitors, wireless printers and routers, and wireless security systems are just a few of the devices we invite into our homes that fill our home with radiation. Radiation can be found in your wireless doorbells, in your home security system, and in any modern car. Our state and national parks now have multiple WiFi antennas; so much for camping and getting away from it all. The most important step to EHS recovery is **avoidance** of EMF. For many, the only way *to not* be affected by radiation is to avoid it all together, which is sometimes impossible in our so-called advanced world. In avoiding EMF, in creating a safe home environment for yourself, you will enjoy renewed health and the ability to better withstand the onslaught of EMF in public.

Decision, Determination and Cooperation

Once you have decided to clean your home of radiation, it takes fortitude to make it happen. This is not an easy project. If you live by yourself, this might come easier than to also convince your partner or living companions of the need. It is amazing how reliant we have become on wireless conveniences. It might seem overwhelming, but be determined. It is more difficult to help your family if you yourself are fighting health issues. In cleaning your home of microwave radiation, you are creating a safe place, a "white zone," a refuge for yourself and family. Respect your health, be strong, as this is an important step to healing, and to accomplish a healing space, **you need an understanding, committed household**.

Sadly, it is not possible to have your wireless handheld device, your wireless routers, and all your wireless conveniences and not have radiation. You either have wireless and radiation or you have wired and no EMF radiation. Once you start looking for wireless devices, you might be confronted with how many radiating devices we rely on. In order to get rid of the radiation associated with them, they need to be wired or unplugged. This doesn't mean you have to do without conveniences, just get them with a wire. Five years ago, it would not have been difficult to clean up a home from wireless. Now, many of our appliances/devices are difficult to find in a wired option, like printers and routers. A suggestion is to plug them in only when in use. I love my computer; it is wired. My phones are corded.

Look at every aspect of your home, from security, wireless music systems, lighting, A/C thermostats, all communications, and everything related to computer and entertainment. The radiating devices in your bedroom could be what are keeping you from sleeping. The popular TV boxes, or anything that streams, emits radiation.

If you discover that you feel fine when away from home, it is time to suspect your own home. If you look around your home or workplace, you'll find that there are many useful conveniences that we take for granted, which rely on radiation. They blend into your décor and you really don't think about them. They might sit in your purse or crouched in a corner; you don't feel them so they are virtually invisible. Remember, anything that streams, emits radiation. A cordless phone emits huge amounts of radiation, but is seldom seen as a possible health threat.

Using Technology Safely

Now that you are aware of what emits radiation, how do you protect yourself?

1. First, get rid of your cordless DECT (digital-enhanced cordless technology) phones. A DECT phone works with a landline, has a base station, handsets and is filling your house with radiation whether it is in use or not. Eric and I have found that DECT phones give off more radiation than many cell phones. At our old home, after we eradicated all wireless devices, the highest radiation we read on our meter came from the neighbor's DECT phone in their kitchen. If you have a landline in your home, don't convert it to wireless. I recommend simply get rid of the cordless phone and replace it with a corded wired phone. If your only phone is a cell phone, consider buying an inexpensive corded phone so you can reduce the radiation they emit.

2. Wireless WiFi routers and wireless printers emit radiation. If it is not possible to have a wired router or printer, it is best to install them well away from where you spend most of your time. The router should definitely not be located in your bedroom, and it is best turned off at night. It is best to purchase routers or printers that do not have wireless capability, as they tend to default to wireless whether you use it with a cord or not. The only way I have found to truly tell if the router is in wireless mode, is with a radiation meter.
3. If an appliance is labeled "smart" in the description, it usually emits EMF through a WiFi signal.
4. Baby monitors should not be used as they equate to a radio station in your baby's room. If you must have some type of monitor, it would be better to use a hardwired security camera in its place, or if not possible, move the child closer to your bed.
5. Dimmer switches are notorious for generating dirty electricity. We changed ours to a standard switch when we moved into our home.
6. Do not keep activated (turned on) wireless devices in your bedroom at night or use your cell phone as an alarm clock.
7. Do not stand by a microwave oven when in use. Distance is your friend. My doctors in Europe told us that "no one should have a microwave oven in their home, period."
8. It would be best to avoid all wireless devices and those you have, turn off when not in use. Evaluate all wireless devices you have and decide how you can best limit their use, if not replace all together with a wired device. This site shown below offers instructions on how to wire an iPad or a cell phone: www.emfanalysis.com/how-to-wire-an-ipad Grounding a wireless laptop with an USB

ground wire does not make it "wired". If it is wireless, it gives off radiation.
9. I believe all children should be kept away from and/or shielded from wireless devices. I believe that pregnant women should wear protective clothing for their growing and sensitive fetus. Online search "EMF protective clothing and shielding."
www.kaiserpermanente.org/article/new-kaiser-permanente-study-provides-evidence-of-health-risks-linked-to-electromagnetic-field-exposure
10. If you have insomnia, you might consider not using your computer/ipad/notebook for several hours before bed, and again, always remove wireless devices from your bedroom.
11. For your wired devices, you might consider putting them on a timer so they turn off automatically in the evening when they would no longer be in use anyway.

Though you clean your home of wireless, you might not feel immediate relief. You might give the changes you made a **trial period** of at least a week; note if you are able to sleep better or your symptoms lessen. I don't know if it was due to the frequency or the amount of radiation I received, but it took me several months to start seeing a difference, and about eight months to feel more like myself. If you do not see a difference after a couple weeks of cleaning your home of radiation, I would advise you to get a radiation meter. It may be that what you are feeling is being introduced from an outside source. The radiation meter would tell you where this outside source emanates and help you eliminate the pollution. After taking steps to stop the radiation, your EMF radiation meter will tell you if you succeeded. (See the chapter on our experiences with EMF radiation meters).

Unless you are someone who can feel the EMFs immediately in many varied situations, a radiation meter is the only way to know that an area will make you ill. One of the best ways to know the source of and avoid radiation is to **carry a radiation meter and use it**. Your EMF meter is the best way to find what is making you ill and help you take steps to mitigate the issues.

Protecting your Home from Outside EMF Sources

You might discover that the radiation in your home is EMF intrusion from an outside source. Visit www.antennasearch.com so that you are aware of the cell towers emitting EMF in the area of your home, work, or places you plan to shop or visit. One of the largest contributors of radiation in your home could be your neighbor's wireless devices. Speak to your neighbors about your issue and you might be able to agree on solutions. You could take the course of offering to pay for wires for your neighbor's router or offending device. We paid for a wired X-box to replace our neighbor's wireless game. If this is not an option open to you, there are quite a few great EMF shielding products, but as of now retail stores do not offer shielding supplies. Following are some suggested solutions and products to keep outside influence of radiation out of your home.

- Paint the inside walls of your home with special high-frequency shielding paint, utilize metalized wallpapers, protective foils, or mesh. Safe Living Technologies (SLT) www.slt.co.
- Window films are also available and work not only on home windows, but we have lined our vehicle windows (see Protective Shelters chapter). We purchased this film from Safe Living Technologies Inc. It is referred to as "Signal Protect Clear".
- Sometimes it is just a simple step, as putting in metal window screens over windows or attaching a piece of metal window screen over a section of wall to solve a 'hot spot'. (Any hardware store should carry aluminum screen.)

- You can apply copper wire mesh or even aluminum window screen on the outside of your home, supported by wood frame from ground to eaves. Be sure to have an overlap of mesh on each side of about 2 inches.
- EMF protection material can be used to line curtains. www.aaronia.com/products/shielding-creening/Aaronia-Shield-50dB

Your radiation meter will tell you if you have solved the problem; your lessening of EHS symptoms will prove it. If you find that your home still has radiation intrusion, you are still feeling ill, outside of a move to a different home, I would suggest building a **Faraday Cage**. (See the chapter Protective Shelters on building a Faraday Cage). There are fabric Faraday shelters at www.LessEMF.com and at Safe Living Technologies. In this way, at least you might sleep uninterrupted and your body may recuperate from its daily abuse of radiation. This would hopefully carry you until you are able to better shield your living space or as a last resort, move. In looking for a new home, so as to know where cell towers were already placed, we used www.antennasearch.com. (We have found recently that not all cell towers are registered or listed.)

Protection from Smart Meter

The radiation energy from a smart meter is delivered in short extreme bursts that are disbursed in all directions. It is gathering information from your home and sending it to a master utility meter located somewhere in your neighborhood. The readings are so high and so fast that some EMF meters cannot read the bursts. As it is radiation, it goes through walls and into your home.

First, I would take steps to opt-out of the smart utility meter if at all possible. I filled out their forms, wrote letter of intent to deny, provided a reason, and attached a copy of my doctor's diagnosis. If you can not opt-out of the smart meter, there are steps one might take that would help to reduce your exposure. If the meter is on the side of your home, it is important to apply shielding between you and the meter. Some find that the utility meter is situated on the wall on the other side of a bed. Knowing that radiation goes through walls, it is crucial to apply shielding between the utility meter and your room. Put metal mesh or metal screening on the wall on both sides, if possible. If you can't move your bedroom to a different room, then you might be able to move the bed to a different wall. Also, many cover the exterior of their smart meter with a metal mesh EMF protective cover that can be purchased on Amazon. Just type in "smart meter" and a myriad of protective RF shielding options are presented. For help with Smart Meter issues: www.emfsafetynetwork.org or www.stopsmartmeters.org

Building Biologist

If you don't feel competent to mitigate the EMFs in your home, there are professional consultants in the business. Building Biology Ecology Consultant (BBEC) and Electromagnetic Radiation Specialist (EMRS) provide assessments that will detect, measure, and reduce sources of EMF radiation in your home, office, or business. They not only test, but offer suggestions and help you clean up your home and know the best products to use for protection. If you can afford it, I would recommend it. If you find that you do not have an available building biologist locally, educate yourself. YouTube is a great source. Read or get on a chat line and learn how others are able to live safely. www.es-forum.com

Why a Radiation Meter is Important

There are instances when I don't immediately recognize I am in an unsafe area. I know that sometimes I feel well, and ten minutes later it feels like the worse case of flu I've ever experienced. There have been occasions where I feel fine, don't suffer ill effects, but experience a delayed reaction putting me in bed for two days. For this reason, I've learned to always carry my radiation meter, so I don't suffer consequences I could have avoided. I would rather be safe than sorry. (See the chapter on EMF Meters.)

Eric and I have several EMF meters, and our favorite as of this writing is the Safe and Sound Pro, purchased through Safe Living Technologies, www.SLT.co. I have found it very important to own a radiation meter and find I use it all the time. For my own health, I have to basically "live by the meter." I have no idea why I don't feel all EMFs right away, and I don't know why I don't always get the same reaction. If I was able to have the same reaction or symptoms—for example, always a migraine headache, or always a stomach ache—then I would be prepared physically, mentally and could possibly pre-medicate for that symptom. It seems each store has their own frequencies, as I get different symptoms in different buildings. For instance, I know that Target Stores always give me head squeezing feeling, confusion, and tunnel vision. I know that our local supermarket always makes me feel like I have the flu, immediately, with hot flashes and nausea. Those two stores are always the same, always immediate. I learned after walking into those stores a few times that I would always be ill upon entering. I also know that there are some stores where I don't feel ill for ten minutes or more; it sneaks up on me. Sometimes I don't feel ill until that evening or the next day. The meter helps immensely by alerting me to EMF dangers. There is no use in feeling ill when I can look at the meter and know I can not go into an area.

The radiation meter can also be a curse. It is the bad guy that says you have to leave when you want to stay. I can enter an area I want to be in, pretend for a minute that I am normal, until I realize that I can't speak or understand what anyone is saying, or I can look at the meter and leave before I feel ill or embarrass myself. I am sure that the meter has saved me many sleepless nights or illness, just by telling me to get out before any damage was done.

Less Radiation at Work

This is, I am sure, a huge challenge for those with EHS that must work. Like your home, you have to be aware of the wireless devices. But what if your employment is in an area of high outside EMF that penetrates the building? Are there clients coming in with their wireless phones and laptops? Does the business require wireless devices for maintenance, inventory, and security? If you are not in charge of the facility, the ways to protect yourself from EMF might be limited.

If you have an open-minded employer or are self-employed, you could limit some exposure by wiring any devices that are close to your work area, including phones. If your desk is close to the wireless router, you could have the router placed in a different location or shield yourself from it by using sheets of aluminum or copper or an inexpensive aluminum window screen as a barrier. You could also try moving your desk farther away. If it is permissible and not a safety issue, you might be consider wearing EMF protective clothing.

Keep a Journal

You might consider keeping a journal of symptoms showing dates and times, as I did. I might not remember if I felt better after the first day or first week after wireless devices were removed, if not for the journals I kept. It is a good idea to keep a diary or journal of when/where you experience symptoms. In this way, a pattern develops that might enlighten you to which areas, stores, or people you have to steer clear of. You may only get symptoms when you enter certain stores, or you may find the skin rash you have disappears when you leave work for vacation. Keeping a diary of symptom days and times would make you more aware of situational symptoms. When you find an area that seems to make you feel ill, stay away for a couple days to see if you get to feeling better. We make it a habit to periodically test our home, work environment, and immediate neighborhood with an EMF meter. This is especially important if you have children you need to protect. We mark readings on a calendar to give us an idea of when or if things change. Environmental changes relating to EMF happen quickly with the advent of so many utilities now using smart meters and neighbors purchasing new EMF emitting devices.

I also keep a file of receipts showing money spent on the EMF shielding products we purchase, just in case they are tax deductible. We have also taken videos of radiation readings showing what the EMF levels. This helps if the readings increase suddenly and you need evidence.

Learn All You Can

The more you learn about EMFs and Electromagnetic Sensitivity, the better you can protect yourself and your family. There are not only many reputable sites that have links to peer-reviewed scientific and medical research papers, but sites that offer help, chat rooms, and articles. There is always something new, everyday, being found in medical breakthroughs and one must know how to search. I have listed some of my favorite websites that specialize in the latest information regarding EMF in the More Information chapter. Here are a couple:

www.CellphoneTaskForce.org
www.MagdaHavas.com
www.MDSafeTech.org

Protect yourself from those who would try to negate how you feel and what you believe. It is difficult to be your own advocate for a malady such as EHS. There are some that do not believe that radiation is harmful. There are some that confuse natural radiation from the sun and earth with man made pulsed non-ionizing radiation. Most don't feel EMF radiation, so don't believe that you could. The worst for me are narrow-minded scientists I speak with who are convinced that because they worked with radiation and they feel fine, I should also. I know how I feel. I know how I became sensitive, and I know I am the evidence. We, the EHS survivors, are the evidence, and we have thousands of knowledgeable physicians that have given our symptoms validity. Do not let an industry shill tell you how you feel. There are syndicated writers whose sole job is to write on behalf of telecommunications industry to hide or downplay the ill-effects of EMF. There are thousands of scientific peer-reviewed reports showing negative health effects of EMF wireless radiation. I am not here to convince anyone of EHS, but rather to help those who find themselves in my situation. If someone doesn't believe, I'm good with that. They can write their own book on how I am wrong.

Stay strong. You are your own best advocate.
EHS support group: www.es-forum.com

Cell Phones and How to Reduce Radiation

Prior to our moving in Germany, our family used a cell phone regularly. Currently, we do have a cell phone, but it is always off unless needed for a flat tire or other emergencies. A cell phone is a convenience that we no longer feel comfortable using due our new found knowledge. For those who find they do not have the option of a wired phone and must depend on their cell phone, there are things you can do to limit your radiation exposure.

1. Minimize wireless phone use, and when possible, use a corded land line. Never hold a cell phone to your head. Either use an air tube headset or the speaker function.

2. Know your cell phone and **how to turn it off** or put on airplane mode. (Note: Some new phones still put out EMFs when on airplane mode, and must be turned off to stop emissions.)

3. Hold your phone away from yourself when turning it on and off, as the phone ramps up energy to "ping" the cell tower. Text messages give off less RF than speaking into your phone/sending. Make your calls short in duration. Also, be aware that many cell phones give off much more RF than they claim.

4. Do not keep the phone on your body, turning off or airplane mode when not in use. Distance is your friend.

5. When carrying a cell phone, it would be wise to not keep it on your person. Never put a cell phone in your bra, by your heart, or in your pants. It would be prudent to

purchase an EMF pocket protector, as they do offer some protection from your phones radiation.

6. Do not use your phone in an area with poor reception or in a vehicle that is not equipped with an exterior antenna. Poor reception makes your phone ramp up the radiation emitted.

7. 4G cell tower vs WiFi. If you must rely on a cell phone at home and you also have WiFi, switching your phone to connect to the WiFi can significantly reduce the phone's radiation output. In tests we performed with a Samsung Galaxy 7 smart phone, the radiation was reduced from 77 $\mu W/m^2$ down to 5 $\mu W/m^2$ by simply connecting to a local WiFi. This is a huge drop in exposure, as the phone is no longer having to connect to a far off 4G cell tower. This reduction occurred while having a conversation, but similar reductions are also seen when transferring data.

8. WiFi Enable. Again, if you must have your phone on, turning it to WiFi enable or WiFi calling will automatically direct your connection to the nearest WiFi, that is if the local WiFi connection is stronger than 4G tower. In this way, your phone is connected through the local WiFi, is still able to ping the 4G tower, but emitting less radiation to do so.

Cell phones vary the radiation they emit, increasing output by as much as ten times depending on the quality of reception to the nearest tower. Try not to use your cell phone in your vehicle as the metal doors and roof can block signal and cause the phone to increase output. This also applies to having your phone on in areas with poor or no cell reception or in metal buildings. When in such areas, it is simply best to turn off the phone. When this is done, you will significantly reduce your exposure, as well as greatly improve your phone's battery life.

"PhoneGate" Cell phone radiation scandal –"After a court filing, the National Frequency Agency (ANFR) of France has just disclosed that most cell phones exceed government radiation limits when tested the way they are used, next to the body. Manufacturers are not required to test phones in shirt or pants pockets. French government tests on hundreds of cell phones reveal that in 2015, 9 out of 10 phones exceed the manufacturer's reported radiation test levels when re-tested in positions where the phone is in contact with the body. The government had refused to disclose these test results until pressure after the court action." https://ehtrust.org/cell-phone-radiation-scandal-french-government-data-indicates-cell-phones-exposeconsumers-radiation-levels-higher-manufacturers-claim/

The FCC radiation limits were designed for safety with a one-time, half-hour exposure. These outdated Specific Absorption Rate or SAR limits were first decided upon in 1996, and only with thermal effects and not biological impacts. Many phones exceed the FCC limit of 1.6 watts per kilogram (1.6 W/kg), and if you'd like to see results of various phones, here is a list compiled by a group in France, where the limit is even higher than in the U.S., at 2 W/kg. Included in the list are American cell phones as well as many used only in Europe. If your phone is not on the list, it doesn't mean that it is deemed safe; it means it wasn't tested. There are three lists: for exposure on the skin, the trunk, and the arms and legs.
https://www.phonegatealert.org/en/check-if-your-mobile-phone-presents-a-risk-to-your-health

I do not believe that there is anything wrong with phones or connecting with others, but we need to be able to limit radiation exposure. Don't be a slave to your cell phone. For those who believe they might want to experience a break from the phone, check out www.catherine-price.com/how-to-break-up-with-your-phone. Be more aware of your surroundings. Celebrate the people you are with by giving them your whole attention. Engage. Look them in the eyes. When you are connected to your phone, you are disconnected with your living life; a piece of you is missing from the "be here, be now." Experience your life.

A Little Information on Cell Phone Health Risk

Effects of the exposure to mobile phones on male reproduction: a review of the literature. www.ncbi.nlm.nih.gov/pubmed/21799142.

The results showed that human spermatozoa exposed to RF-EMR have decreased motility, morphometric abnormalities, and increased oxidative stress, whereas men using mobile phones have decreased sperm counts, decreased motility (particularly rapid progressive motility), normal morphology, and decreased viability. These abnormalities seem to be directly related to the duration of mobile phone use.

Scientists in Korea have additionally found something called "digital dementia" children. They reported that children who are heavy technology users have brains that are under-developed on the right side. This has been characterized by memory loss, attention disorders, lack of eye contact, lack of empathy, and difficulty feeling or showing emotions. As a result, the Korean government is instituting programs to reduce usage and exposures especially to young children.

"In summary, there is reasonable basis to conclude that RF-EMFs are bioactive and have a potential to cause health impacts. There is a consistent pattern of increased risk for glioma and acoustic neuroma associated with use of wireless phones (mobile phones and cordless phones) mainly based on results from case-control studies from the Hardell group and Interphone Final Study results. Epidemiological evidence gives that RF-EMF should be classified as a human carcinogen. The current safety limits and reference levels are not adequate to protect public health. New public health standards and limits are needed." Use of Mobile Phones and Cordless Phones is Associated with Increased Risk for Glioma and Acoustic Neuroma, www.emfsafetynetwork.org/wp-content/uploads/2013/10/Cell-and-Cordless-Phones-risk-for-cancer.pdf

EMF Meters and ELF Meters

Section written by Eric Mills

During the poisoning event, it was not possible to determine the highest radiation levels measured, as they exceeded what the measuring equipment could read. The report reads a minimum of 20,000,000 micro watts per square meter ($\mu W/m^2$) were recorded, with a note that the situation on site suggests multiples of this level. Numerous locations at the home recorded readings of 10,000,000 $\mu W/m^2$ and above, which were within the equipment's capabilities. The readings taken at our home represent peak microwave power. It is important to understand the difference between "peak power" and "average power". Time averaged measurement of power is the result of industry's opinion that all that matters with non-ionizing radiation are thermal effects, and averaged energy levels is what affects heating. However, most wireless devices spend a large proportion of time sporadically transmitting. This is why you want to read peak levels, not average. Many hundreds of studies have documented non-thermal adverse health effects of these frequencies and the measurement of peak signal strength is more applicable when equating complex digitally modulated, non-continuous signals with ill-effects on individuals. This is why we utilize our meter's peak power readings measured in volts per meter (V/m) in determining what exposure levels adversely impact Anne.

Radiation Meters

Electrosmog Analyzer HF35C

We purchased our first radiation meter after returning to California from Germany in 2009. It was an Electrosmog Analyzer HF35C, made by Gigahertz Solutions in Germany and purchased through Safe Living Technologies, Inc. The meter was expensive, high quality, and equipped with a large Christmas tree looking directional antenna. The meter has a sound function, and once familiar with the sounds, I could differentiate between Cell Phones, WiFi networks, Smart Meters, cordless home phones, etc. In using our radiation meter, we were shocked at the many sources of EMF we were being exposed to and surrounded by. Where we had been solely focusing on cell towers, we became increasingly aware of our neighbors' WiFi and cordless home phones. The emissions of these wireless devices could expose you to significantly higher levels of EMF than far distant cell towers, because of their closer proximity!

In 2011, we moved to a quiet country setting, three hours from the populated Bay Area. Upon returning from a vacation back to our rural country home that had been free of EMF, Anne felt that something had changed. We checked our Gigahertz meter and it didn't show any EMF in the house. One key limitation of this first meter was its narrow bandwidth of 800 MHz to 2.5 GHz, which failed to include many higher frequencies that were now increasingly used by the wireless industry. I quickly reassembled the Faraday Shelter last used in the Bay Area to give Anne protection and purchased a new meter with a broader range of frequencies.

Cornet brand meter (ED85EXS)

I chose a Cornet brand meter (ED85EXS) with frequencies ranging from 700 MHz up to 6 GHz. Upon its delivery, this new tool showed us that there was, in fact, EMF in our home. Using the new meter, I was able to trace the source to our neighbor's house about 150 feet away. The source of the EMF was our neighbor's brand new remote control for their Nintendo X-Box video game! Our neighbors were well aware of Anne's EHS and had fought off installation of a "smart meter" on their house in consideration of her health. Here we had an instance where neither they nor we had any idea that a wireless hand control could cause an issue. We purchased a wired X-Box for their use, and once the wireless hand control was disconnected, all radiation stopped. Anne was out of the Faraday cage again.

Cornet brand (Model MD18)
Our next meter was a higher end Cornet brand (Model MD18) that has many more functions than the previous meter's basic functions and a wider range of frequencies from 100MHZ to 8 GHz. It has an internal antenna that makes it much less conspicuous when in use out in public. The unit displays power density, frequencies, and has a nice hysteresis screen that shows the previous thirty readings. We find the hysteresis helpful, as sometimes Anne walks through an area where she feels EMF and this function allows us to review just how high those levels were. We did find that these meters are fragile, as we had to order a second meter (same model MD18) because I dropped and broke the first one. These last meters served us well and we found that we became reliant on them in determining if an area was safe for Anne to be in.

Acoustimeter (Model AM10)
Over time, we found that Anne could sense EMF even though the meters were reading nothing! This lead us to an EMFields-brand Acoustimeter. This meter can read frequencies 200 Mhz to 8 Ghz. Although high in quality, it is quite basic when compared to the multi-function Cornet. It has no back light screen, no frequency counter, no hysteresis, but it shows the presence of EMF that the Cornet failed to read. Anne hated it when we first got it, as it showed places that Anne thought were safe and free of EMF that actually were not. The Acoustimeter has sound just like our first meter where you can hear the distinctive buzz, hiss, and rhythmic clicks of various sources, even if the signals are very faint. We've learned to be very careful with our meters and now carry it in a nice padded pouch with a shoulder strap. Anne carries the meter with the sound

function turned up so she can immediately become aware of sources of radiation that may have entered her surroundings.

The users' manual for our Acoustimeter states that few people report ill-effect from readings below 0.05 volts per meter (V/m), some individuals report ill-effects between 0.05 and 0.5 V/m and that nearly all sensitive individuals report experiencing adverse health effects above 0.5 V/m. This means that Anne is slightly more sensitive than what the user's manual states.

A new lower cost alternative is now available in the Acousticom 2, which costs under $200 and offers the same wide range of frequencies and peak power readings, but without average power readings.

Safe and Sound Pro

We just recently purchased the Safe and Sound Pro when we found radiation in our home that none of our meters could read. We suspected that the new exposures were from frequencies higher than the 8 Ghz that our Acoustimeter could detect. The Safe and Sound Pro can effectively read frequencies as high as 12 GHz. We learned that this meter has a greater level of accuracy than the Acoustimeter at higher frequencies. The meter is simple to use and smaller in size than the Acoustimeter. The meter is easier to use at night as it has an illuminated display with four lights indicating slight, moderate, high, and extreme levels of RF. However, the meters sound function is not nearly as loud as the Acoustimeter. The Safe and Sound Pro reads peak levels in microwatts per square meter $\mu W/m^2$, as opposed to V/m. This meter comes in a nice protective case and reasonably priced at approximately $400. We have also found that Safe Living Technologies in Canada offer high quality products and provide great service and technical advice. www.slt.co

With the advent of 5G, we will still not have a meter that can detect the EMF emitted. Currently there is no meter available for under $5000 able to read the very high millimeter wave-length frequencies that true 5G will emit.

How much radiation is too much?

Through trial and error, we have found that an environment of >0.20 Volts per Meter (V/m) for any period of time is too much for Anne, as she starts experiencing discomfort, loss of vocabulary, etc. As an example, this level is significantly lower than the average person is exposed to if they carry a smart phone or have a WiFi router in their home.

Another key take-away with our use of radiation meters is the massive exposure levels we see while traveling. We observe readings on the freeway greater than our Acoustimeter can read (>6.0 V/m.) If you can see a cell tower along the road side, you are being exposed to extreme levels of radiation. Our meter can also measure RF Power Density, which is measured in micro-watts per square meter ($\mu W/m^2$). Although our meter can read levels to 100,000 $\mu W/m^2$, we have driven through areas that exceed these readings for minutes on end. This led to us to take steps to shield our vehicle. (See the Protective Shelters chapter).

Where we now live, the closest cell tower is about fourteen miles away, with many hills and valleys that result in poor or no cell phone signal strength. We've learned that cell phones ramp up their energy as they try to communicate with the nearest cell tower. This can be as high as a factor of ten times the radiation emitted depending on the signal strength, and is the reason the battery life on a cell phone is so short when traveling through a rural countryside. These high levels of radiation also happen when using your phone in your car, as the vehicle acts as a Faraday Cage. Your phone is forced to ramp up energy in order to communicate with the tower. You are being exposed to high levels of radiation in your car, whenever your phone is on, and not even being utilized.

Dirty Electricity and ELF Meters

Through our interaction with experts in the field, we have subsequently learned of risks from extreme-low frequencies (ELF). ELF or dirty electricity is "when the electrical power lines and wiring within your home contain frequencies other than the normal 60 Hz electrical current (50 Hz in Europe). These additional frequencies piggyback on the electrical wiring and radiate into your living environment. These frequencies then interact with your body." (From www.emfanalysis.com). ELF can cause negative health effects similar to that of electromagnetic frequencies from wireless devices.

Graham Stetzer Meter / Filters.
As the hum of neon lights didn't seem to adversely impact Anne, we hadn't really looked into this as an issue. As a precaution, we did take steps to minimize ELF or dirty electricity in our home. We bought a small kit that contained a Graham Stetzer Meter and eight Graham Stetzer Filters. Using the meter, we first measured dirty electricity levels at all of the electrical outlets in the house and then applied filters to those circuits with the highest readings on the meter. The guidelines on the instructions that come with the kit, state that the circuits should ideally be less than 20 Graham Stetzer units (GS) and best to never exceed 50 GS units as shown on meter. We found that most of our outlets read approximately 150 GS. One filter in that circuit is usually enough to achieve the desired lower readings. This action significantly reduced, or filtered out the dirty frequencies throughout our home.

A later event did seem to indicate that Anne is, in fact, adversely affected by high levels of ELF. Solar Voltaic cells were installed on the roof of our local community center where she spends time as a volunteer. Anne had not known that these newly-installed solar panels had been activated when she had to cut short a visit to the center complaining of severe headaches and a heaviness like "wearing a heavy pot" on her head. Later that same day I took the Stetzer Meter into the community center and measured huge levels of dirty electricity (>2000 GS!) in the very area that she spent the most time. It turns out that the cheap inverters typically used by the solar power industry generate high levels of dirty electricity that permeate throughout the entire building to which they are connected. We found that all we needed to eliminate this new source of ELF was to apply Stetzer Filters on the outlets in the room that Anne is in. So the new routine is whenever Anne is going to the center, she gathers up six filters from home and places them around the electrical outlets in the community hall.

    Just recently, Anne was having a poor night's sleep every time we visited our travel trailer. We had previously tested the trailer for the presence of dirty electricity and found it to be relatively low. After a second poor night's sleep, she noticed that the one Stetzer filter in the trailer was making a faint buzzing noise. I decided to recheck the ELF levels and found huge levels were in fact present. We had recently started to use a small electrical heater in the bathroom of the trailer at night, as fall was setting in and the overnight temperatures were getting colder. Once I unplugged this new heater, all the buzzing stopped and the meter readings fell to acceptable levels. We got rid of that heater and Anne hasn't had a bad night's sleep since. We had no idea a little electric heater could cause such a problem.

    With further research, we discovered that dirty electricity is a huge issue for many people. No matter the source, be it external power lines or an internal source of these transients, the Stetzer Filters seem to effectively eliminate these harmful frequencies. CFL Light Bulbs and dimmer switches can also present a significant source of transient ELF, so we simply don't use them. For those sensitive to dirty electricity, there are many sites with information on how to protect your home.

Anne Mills

www.EmfAnalysis.com/what-is-dirty-electricity
www.emfacademy.com/dirty-electricity-dangerous/
www.electricsense.com/10088/dirty-electricity-dave-stetzer

TriField EMF Meter

We just bought a new TriField EMF meter that can measure not only RF frequencies that all our previous meters have measured, but it can also read AC Magnetic and AC Electrical (dirty electricity) energies.

I am sure with as fast as technology changes, there will be many new meters made available that will be more affordable with a broader range of EMF spectrum. I wish you best of luck in your purchases. I have included photos of our array of meters.
Eric Mills

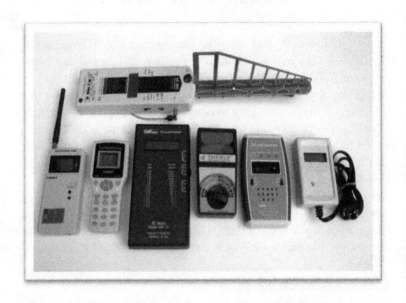

Top
Electrosmog Analyzer HF35C, with directional antenna

Bottom, Left to Right
Cornet brand meter (ED85EXS), Cornet brand (Model MD18), Acoustimeter (Model AM10), TriField EMF Meter, Safe and Sound Pro, Graham Stetzer Meter

Situational Awareness

I physically feel invisible electromagnetic field radiation (EMF) in a very real and painful sense. It is difficult to describe or quantify EMF felt during an exposure. Occasionally, it feels like being physically pushed backwards. Other times, it feels like an illness. This is what I try to convey when I explain how much EMF it takes to give one tremors, aches, and nausea. EMFs are easier to evaluate with a radiation meter, but to then equate that number with a pain or discomfort adds another level of difficulty to describe. Everyone has their own level of tolerance. Every person has their own definition of too much. Due to my sensitivities, 0.10 V/m (volts per meter) is about as high as I can tolerate for any length of time. This means that 0.20 V/m is quite uncomfortable and 0.40 V/m is too much and I must leave.

Living by the Meter

The meter tells me if I can be somewhere when I might not have symptoms immediately, and it also validates my feelings if I do sense EMF. When I first enter a questionable area, I think, "Well, maybe I can handle it." I can partake of events for a only a short period before I start feeling ill with headaches, hot flashes, nausea, tunnel vision. Occasionally I've had to leave, apologizing to Eric, whom I am sure has been looking forward to the event. So, not only am I feeling ill, but feeling guilty.

When I begin feeling ill, I tend to not think of Electromagnetic Sensitivity (EHS) as the first issue. When I first feel an EMF exposure I exhibit a bad case of denial and second guess myself. I start wondering if I did not drink enough water or am possibly coming down with the flu, or think I should have eaten before venturing out. EHS symptoms, for me at least, appear different in different situations. Sometimes my symptoms are delayed, and occasionally don't become evident at all until evening or the next morning. Following are a few situations explaining why it is prudent to live by the meter.

Last summer we went camping with a local camping club. We had entered the address into www.antennasearch.com and found no cell towers listed close to the campground. We prepared our gear and headed out looking forward to a vacation. When we arrived, our meters were showing that the whole campgrounds EMF measurements were extremely high (over >3.0 V/m). There were only two campsites in the entire park low enough for us to set up camp, (<0.20 V/m) and luckily, they were vacant. I found that the radiation was too high to walk around the campground or even saunter to the river. What was going on? We had no idea that the campground was located right by a Coast Guard station, which obviously utilizes a huge amount of radio and cell equipment. Thank goodness, the van was shielded or I would not have lasted the night. We thought we had done our homework in looking for nearby cell antenna, only to learn we needed to look for government services that might greatly pollute with EMF. We were glad we only lived about four hours away, as we could only stay one night. We were happy our plan B includes carrying an EMF-protective sleeping bag.

***

Having lived in Bavaria, we had come to love beer festivals. After moving back to the U.S., we thought we'd take in an October Beer Fest in Oregon. As we knew it was a long push and if anything happened we could not make it home in one day, we not only investigated how near to the campsites the cell towers were located, but also how close the cell towers were to the festival. (www.antennasearch.com) We booked two campsites, one by the festival, and as a plan B, one at a secluded campsite about half an hour out of town. The beer fest was just getting started, and we had volunteered to pour beer in one of the tents. We were all dressed in our *lederhosen*. Upon arriving and checking the different venues with our meters, all hopes were dashed when we found the radiation was extremely high (>4.5 V/m) in the main tent. There was no way I could be in there with my sensitivity. It turns out that one side of the beer tent was near the town's water tower, which was rimmed with WiFi antenna. We walked around the festival testing all the different venues, and found one where the EMFs were low (<0.20 V/m) as this area was it was in the shadow of a steel-sided warehouse. We were able to stay in this area all day! It did mean, however, that the campsite at the festival had radiation readings that were exorbitant and were so glad we had made plan B reservations or we would not have had a place to stay for the night.

***

We traveled to Death Valley, to meet a friend at the campsite and surprise him for his birthday. We found and made camp only to find that the radiation was extremely high (>4.5 V/m) from the WiFi and cell phone towers around Furnace Creek. We left the next day. Beware in traveling to the Death Valley, as driving through an adjoining military base peaked our meter (>6.0 V/m) inside our van, even with the EMF protective window tinting. Yikes. We have found that the best camping is remote camping, where there are no utilities and the sites are large and away from others. Also, if you can afford it, group campsites are good, as you are allotted space between sites.

***

One vacation we booked little cabins along a river that had no cell antenna within five miles and no WiFi onsite. Amazingly, we found high radiation in our room. We found that there was a wireless rodent device plugged in under the bed. Once we unplugged it we had a nice night sleep. One has to take into account that so many devices are wireless, and this rodent deterrent was a new one for us. One should always carry metalized clothing, meters and have a plan B. Travel with EHS is not easy, which is heartbreaking, as I've always loved to travel.

***

The simple act of being in traffic puts Eric and I in a trying situation. I cannot sit in traffic on a freeway without feeling ill. The radiation on freeways is massive, at times peaking the meter (>6.0 V/m) with cell towers and repeaters, many autos with wireless sensors, and every vehicle with a cell phone. Even with our EMF protective window shielding, I begin to feel ill and resort to plan B by putting on my protective clothing. At times this is not enough and we have to turn to plan C, which is to find the nearest exit.

***

Self-reliance is key to the wellbeing of those with EHS. I am afraid that no one else is going to look out for our health and certainly not the government. The Federal Communications Commission (FCC) is a captured agency, influenced and controlled by people that work for, or have close ties to, the wireless industry. The FCC is supposed to be policing and setting limits to protect our welfare and wellbeing. The FCC sells the licenses and sets EMF radiation limits on industry, but their limits date back to 1996 and only take in thermal heating. They know the dangers to the population, but they like the money better. Unlike Europe, here in the U.S. there isn't an agency that monitors whether the lax EMF radiation limits set by the FCC are even adhered to. In the U.S., the wireless industry is self-regulated, meaning there is no department in the government of, by, or for the citizens, protecting the citizens from man-made radiation. The U.S. is putting masts up in massive numbers.

The best way to protect yourself from EMF radiation is to "live by the meter," be prepared with protective clothing, and always have a plan B. Where do you go and how do you protect yourself if your first plans don't work; if it turns out that a new tower or new antenna or a new router has been put in your vicinity? What do you do if someone with a cell phone containing its own hot spot enters your space? Eric and I have had so many instances where we plan, get all excited about an upcoming event, and find that the area is all EMF'd up, the pulsed microwave radiation is so high that it drives us out. So, become aware of EMF sources where you live and where you spend time. Learn areas where it is safe to be and areas you must avoid due to EMF radiation. Always carry around your protective clothing.

    For those who also feel EMF, our bodies are trying to tell us that an area is not safe. As much as we'd like to live in the moment and ignore them, we need to pay attention to our body's warnings. One must always be aware of their surroundings. You can only do this if you are armed with knowledge.

Protective Shelters

Written by Eric Mills

Faraday Shelters

What is a Faraday shelter or Faraday cage? The Faraday cage was invented in 1836 by the English scientist Michael Faraday, known as the "father of electricity." A Faraday cage/shelter is an enclosure used to block electromagnetic fields. It is formed by having a continuous encasement of conductive material, such as wire mesh, surrounding an enclosed space. A microwave oven is a good example of a Faraday cage. The oven's walls, top, bottom, and door are all made of conductive material that shields the radiation from escaping. If you look closely through the oven's door, (not while it is on) you'll see a layer of fine wire mesh that stops the radiation from passing through the glass. A magnetron inside the oven generates microwave frequencies (EMF) that are shielded from escaping. Around the oven door is a magnetic strip that assures a leak-free bond between the door and the oven wall. In our case, we have built a very large metallic cage, or Faraday cage, that we climb into and thus are shielded from external sources of EMF.

The first Faraday cage I constructed was in the attic of our little home in Sophienthal, Germany. We had just moved into this new rental house in the country, but still found that EMF levels at night were too high for Anne. Dr. Eger instructed me on how such a shelter should be built. I constructed the cage in the attic, where entry was gained by a pull-down ladder on the ceiling. It was out of sight to visitors because we did not know how concerned our new landlady would be with its construction. We had read that chicken wire could be used to form a continuous circle of conducting surface. We included a wired panel to lay over the opening of the fold down stairway. This Faraday cage worked very well at shielding out EMF. We were even able to have its effectiveness tested by Herr Wenz with his EMF meter.

It was wonderful to have a safe place for Anne, but the attic space wasn't insulated; very hot in the short German summer and very cold as winter approached. It was difficult going up and down the attic ladder in the middle of the night to go to the bathroom, but we thought the trade-off of convenience for the ability to sleep was positive. Anne looked forward to the cage, as she was so sleep deprived that even climbing into an attic was passable.

With the extreme temperature fluctuation in the attic Faraday cage, I constructed a second cage in our bedroom before winter. It was constructed using the same wire mesh, but made up of interlocking large panels. The panels were wood covered on all sides with the wire. This cage did not work well, and I believe it was due to insufficient continuity between these individual wire mesh sections. This meant that the cage could not hold its own resonance. I also found that the doorway was a critical design element that needed changing. I tried adding more wire mesh to the cage, and even tried sewing the panels together with wire, but to no avail. Although we did not have a radiation meter of our own at this time, Anne could feel that radiation was leaking in.

I constructed a third cage soon after in the basement. This had the added shielding benefit of being partially below ground and this cage worked very well. It was made with the same chicken wire but in continuous loops with each loop overlapping about two inches. This assured complete coverage and conductivity between loops. Being in the basement was also helpful, as when the landlord checked on the condition of her rental, it was disguised behind some storage closets. In fact, we entered the cage through a door of one of the storage cabinets. We were afraid that if the landlady, or anyone, knew we had to sleep in a cage, we might lose our home. (We later learned that the fear was unfounded; our landlady, Heidi, was compassionate and understanding.) In addition, having the door incorporated into the storage cabinet also assured much improved continuity. One key takeaway was that all electronic devices, lights, or alarm clock had to be external to the shelter. As wire mesh was being used, the shelter was not as claustrophobic as the second panel Faraday enclosure had been. This third shelter in Sophienthal served us for the following two years. Most nights we would start out in our bedroom and if Anne would sense radiation we would go down to the cage, as we called it. Many nights, Anne would sense the EMF and we would just start off in the cage.

Fabric Shelter

Once we moved back to California, we found that the EMF levels required a Faraday shelter also. Our return to the United States coincided with the roll-out of smart meters. We purchased a metalized EMF protective fabric shelter to surround our bed through www.lessemf.com. It was made of very fine, woven, transparent veil-like material that extended all around and under the bed, which was designed to be hung from the ceiling. We quickly found that some form of framework was necessary. I built a large box shaped frame around the bed constructed of long 1" by 2" wooden strips and draped the fabric over it. Access was gained by lifting up one side of the veil and climbing under the fabric. This Faraday cage did not seem to work very well shielding out EMF. Also, the act of getting in and out soon contaminated the fabric at the entry point. We made attempts to add grounding wires to increase the effectiveness, and even added clothespins in an attempt to improve conductivity around the side that we climbed into the enclosure. It may be due to Anne's increasing sensitivity, but none of these steps seemed to improve its performance for our situation. For a while, we also tried a white noise machine to help drown out the hum Anne heard, but to no avail.

Anne Mills

Evolving Faraday Design

    With a cell tower being erected in the neighborhood, we were forced to move once more. This new home is where I designed and constructed our final Faraday cage, which we still use. It is a rigid structure incorporating all that we had learned from our past successes and mistakes. Importantly, the entrance to this new cage is built with a very substantial doorway assuring full continuity. The door is actually a separate panel; a "plug" that we insert into the opening once we climb inside. Around this opening and surrounding the plug are strips of metal flashing that assure good electrical continuity. Unlike the cages built in Germany, where we had utilized chicken wire, this new shelter uses four-foot-wide, galvanized quarter-inch hardware cloth, sourced from the local building supply. This cage is a free-standing, box-frame construction, built up around the bed and is large inside. (See Faraday cage pictures) After the initial build, we added grounding wires out the second-story window down to a long grounding bar sunk into the soil. It worked wonderfully! Sadly, with more external sources of EMF, from newly installed smart meters and neighbor's WiFi networks, Anne sometimes needed to stay in the cage all day. Because of this, we moved our household to a much more remote location to escape all the EMFs.

All EMF*d Up

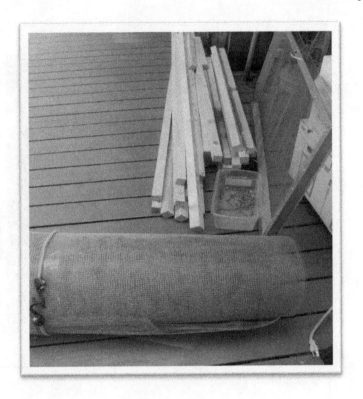

Materials Needed:
- Metal Hardware Cloth
- Wood Two by Two's
- Metal Screws
- Metal Flashing
- Two simple door handles (fixed)

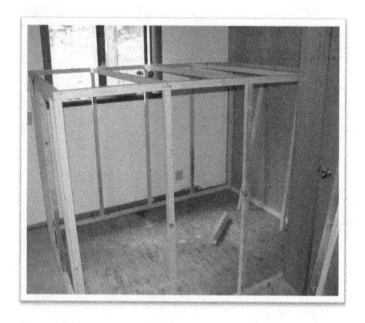

Assemble Frame.

Install wire mesh to floor.

Add bed.

Staple wire mesh to all remaining walls and ceiling, overlapping any seams.

[

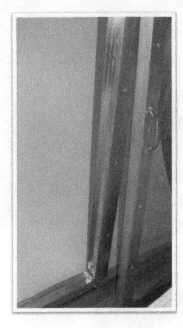

Doorway opening and plug with flashing

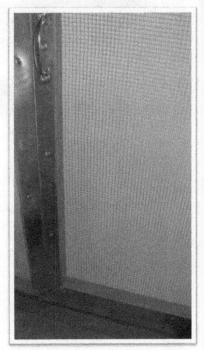

Doorway plug inserted from inside - Tight fit to ensure conductivity.

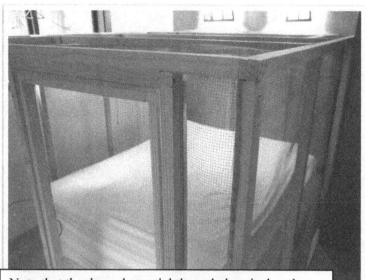

Note that the door closes tightly and electrical outlets and lights are on outside of Faraday Cage

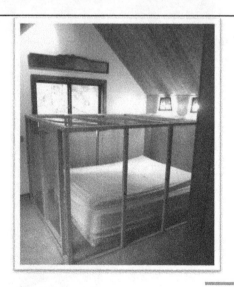

With ever higher frequencies being employed by the wireless industry, ever smaller wire mesh may be required to assure the effectiveness of your Faraday cage. Aluminum screen or even solid foil may be necessary, particularly once 5G is rolled out. The guideline we've used is that the openings of the wire mesh should be no larger than one quarter of the wavelength. http://www.hottconsultants.com/techtips/freq-wavelength.html (More information on Faraday cages can be found if you search for "Faraday cage DIY") Faraday cages are commonly used by industry for testing purposes and for protecting sensitive electronics, and are commonly available through many sources such as Holland Shielding.

We recently found that our home was being exposed at night to a new source of EMF. Our meters showed no radiation, and our Faraday cage was unable to screen out these new frequencies. This forced us out of the house at night, and into our vehicle for protection. We ordered and received a new meter that did detect high levels of radiation which in turn validated the symptoms Anne was experiencing. A test using aluminum screen in front of the new meter showed that it was effective at blocking out these higher the frequencies. This prompted me to immediately apply aluminum screen over the existing hardware cloth used in the Faraday cage. We were now out of our vehicle and back in the house, but having to use the Faraday cage at night.

RF Shielding Foil Faraday

We believe the radiation is getting progressively worse. Anne started feeling EHS symptoms at night, even in the modified shelter, that were quite similar to those she felt in Germany. We purchased a more accurate radiation meter with a broader spectrum of frequencies that showed new microwave energy in our home. It became apparent that I needed to build a new cage, as the aluminum screen that we had added to our Faraday cage did not filter out these new frequencies.

I purchased reflective non-perforated foil material from Safe Living Technologies (www.slt.co). This heavy weight foil comes in rolls four foot wide by 125 feet long, is tear resistant and is easy to cut with just a scissor. I utilized it to construct a new cage by lining the smallest room in our home. This small triangular space is a loft which had held a guest bed. As the foil is highly conductive, I taped over all wall outlets with electrical tape. I attached the material with staples to the floor and all the walls, (see pictures) overlapping the seams by two inches and securing the seams together with metalized tape purchased from same company.

On a Faraday cage, the door is always the most critical. To construct the door, I cut a narrow three-sided flap opening, leaving material attached on the header. I cut a rectangular piece of material several inches wider than the door flap and attached it to the inside with tape. This created an overlap with the foil on either side of the doorway, assuring a tight fit when closed. I taped small magnets on the two vertical sides of the outside of the door opening. When open, the flap is rolled upward and a single piece of duct tape holds this rolled flap open. To close the door we roll down the material and hand place magnets on the inside that correlate to those placed on outside. This assures a tight seal between the doorway and the roll down flap.

This foil material is not breathable at all and it is imperative that you find a way to ventilate the area. This loft space has a small window which is great as it provides outside light and air into this confined space. I put five layers of aluminum window screen over the window to, hopefully, screen out EMF. I used a small portable battery pack that has a cigarette lighter jack, and a portable twelve volt fan made for an auto. Propped in the window, this fan brings fresh air into the space all night. Without the window I would have had to devise a shielded air baffle.

All EMF*d Up

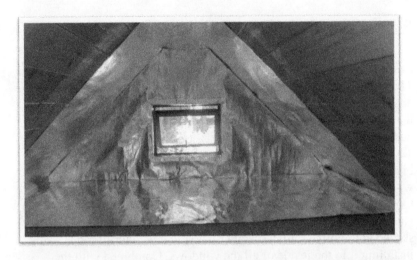

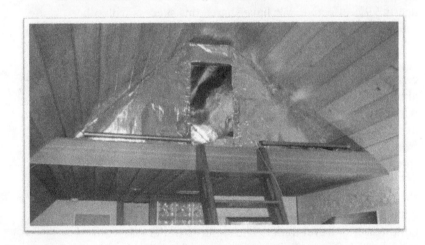

Anne Mills

Rolling Faraday Shelter

Once we moved to our more rural home, our meters showed us that our biggest EMF exposure was while traveling. The readings are surprisingly high when driving past cell towers and through built-up areas. We found a special window tinting that incorporated anti-eavesdropping shielding used by the FBI and State Department. We purchased this film from Safe Living Technologies Inc. It is referred to as "Signal Protect Clear". A big challenge was that this film tinting was made for buildings with flat glass, unlike car window tinting, which is made stretchy to allow it to be applied to curved glass. We purposely bought a van because most of its glass is nearly flat. We found a highly skilled automotive tinting installer who did a wonderful job installing it to the inside of all the windows. Combined with the steel panels on this van, the attenuation has been measured to be nearly 99% effective. We have shared this success with other sensitives and the installer has applied this shielding to a number of other vehicles since.

We had found that when camping, the inside of the van can get very hot with all the windows closed. I recently made aluminum screens cut to the shape of the front passenger door windows that can be easily affixed to the outside of the doors using magnets. These screens now allow us to roll down the front windows while sleeping and still assure that radiation is shielded out.

We have two other examples of a rolling Faraday shelter. In an attempt to travel across the country to see our grandchildren on the East Coast, we purchased a used, custom-built, teardrop travel trailer. The teardrop trailer was skinned entirely with sheets of aluminum except for the underside. We thought this would provide a safe environment for Anne as we camped along the way to the East Coast and back. The teardrop trailer had many shortfalls. It didn't work very well as a Faraday cage, even after we added wire mesh to the underside and shielded fabric for the windows. Numerous times on the trip,

Anne would awaken to find high EMF levels inside the cabin that forced us to break camp and flee. Also, the teardrop trailer was small and not well insulated. Coming into Memphis on a 100-degree day, when we stopped to set up camp along the Mississippi, it was 100 degrees inside the trailer, too! We later sold the teardrop trailer.

The other rolling Faraday shelter is our old 28-foot 1972 travel trailer. It looks very much like an Airstream, all clad in anodized aluminum sheet metal. We've had it long before this EMF poisoning event occurred. We keep the trailer in a small trailer park and see it as a safe place for Anne to just get away; that is until the trailer park installed WiFi. The antenna was pointed directly at our trailer and resulted in huge EMF readings outside with some penetration inside. All turned out well, however, when another camper complained that their trailer spot could not access the WiFi signal and asked if we would swap sites. Moving the trailer reduced the external EMFs significantly, but we were still not totally WiFi free inside. We found EMF leaking in through the windows, which we were able to eliminate by simply applying aluminum window screen. We never travel with this huge trailer, but we now have our safe spot back!

EMF Blocking Sleeping Bag

We purchased a Microwave Protection Sleeping Bag (BlocBag) through LessEMF.com in 2010 as a safety bivouac when traveling. We have used it only a couple of times on our cross-country trip inside the teardrop Trailer. There were places we had camped that initially seemed to have low EMF, that only after setting up camp we discovered were too high for comfort. The BlocBag is a zip-up cocoon, all-encompassing bag, (96 x 34 inch) made from Swiss Shield Wear material for the body portion and Swiss Shield Daylite mesh for the hooded area. Anne thought it was somewhat claustrophobic completely zipped up, but both times she felt thankful that we had it when the EMF levels built up too intense. The bag is only 22dB attenuation below 1.8 GHz, but we always carry it with us in our vehicle just in case we have to stay somewhere we can't control the environment. In our case, we would use the EMF protective sleeping bag in addition to other protection measures.

We consistently observe extremely high EMF radiation readings while in our shielded vehicle. We would recommend that if you are an EHS sufferer you either shield your vehicle or wear personal shielded clothing to be comfortable during travel.

Personal EMF Protection

Once I became cognizant of the full extent of what being Electromagnetic Sensitive (EHS) meant, the first thing that came to mind was how to protect myself. What would protection from invisible electromagnetic fields (EMF) look like and where would I get it? Could I afford protection? When my poisoning occurred, we lived in a rural area and there was no way to protect myself from the cell towers other than moving. Moving is not an option for everyone, and the previous chapters on how to protect your home offer various suggestions. But how does one protect themselves when away from their personal safe White Zone? If home is not totally defensible, what does one use for protection?

The area we now live in does not have a dense population and we also don't have the radiation emissions from small cell antenna. This might not be the case in the future, which would be detrimental to my health. My husband and I could suddenly have new neighbors who enjoy all things wireless, or a cell tower could be erected too close for my wellbeing. Both situations would be life changing. Every day I wonder when the EMF encroachment will hit a critical tipping point. The main way I protect myself is avoidance. When this is not an option, I use protective shielded clothing.

The last few nights I have been experiencing hot flashes, headaches that include jaw pain, and allergy symptoms. I know that these are associated with EMF, as they begin at a set time; exactly at 12:15 am and again at 2:15 am, the energy turning off gradually along with the symptoms. This totally disrupts any attempts for a good night sleep and brings back vivid memories of the past EMF poisoning event in Germany. I do have a Faraday cage that my husband made and I could take refuge there. (See the chapter Protective Shelters.) What would I do if I did not have the cage? I would make immediately call and order EMF protective shielded clothing, at least for my head, or an EMF protective sleeping bag. Lying in bed with metalized cloth

bag on my head or in a sleeping bag is not all that comfortable. There has to be a better way, but I know of none other than a Faraday cage. As the protective clothing might take a couple days for delivery, I would find a friend I could stay with until I was able to mitigate the issue, and hope their EMF situation was better.
(LessEMF.com 1-888-537-7363)

Protective clothing

When we moved back to the states from Germany, we learned that the radiation here in California was prolific. Though avoidance of EMF is the first rule, I realized that EMF protective clothing was imperative in public. I was discovering that the number of places I could safely endure for any length of time was diminishing, one of them being my parents' home. In looking for EMF protective clothing in 2010 there were not many choices on the market. Luckily the online store LessEMF.com had some affordable ready-made clothing available and I purchased their hoody. Now, with an online search, I can find several companies that have joined LessEMF in offering ready-made EMF protective clothing. One can now purchase hoodies, pants, dress shirts, gloves, head protection, undershirts, and socks, among other items.

I had purchased and used hoodies and open-faced head coverings, but continued to experience headaches and vertigo. I started to believe it was the fact that my headgear was open faced. Radiation might be stopped by the metalized material in the back of my head, but what about my face? Did the radiation enter my face and not have a place to disburse? I purchased a full-face EMF protective headgear, and for me the problem disappeared. I no longer was ill within a short ten-minute EMF exposure. I now only wear full-faced head protection. This got me to think about the aprons that are offered for women who are pregnant and only cover their belly. Pregnant women might want to consider wearing protection that doesn't just protect the front, but their back also.

Due to the proliferation of, and increase in, EMF radiation and my negative reaction to them, I realized that I needed something that covered my whole body and not just my head. I do not know about other EHS survivors, but I found myself becoming more sensitive. The biggest wake-up call was when I found that due to the massive EMF at the cemetery, I could not attend my father's funeral or memorial. The EMF made me ill before the service even started. This was a sad way to discover I needed clothing that had more attenuation, or radiation protective qualities.

Eric found new improved metalized materials on the European market. In Europe, metalized material is a bit more expensive and one must purchase it by linear meter, not the yard. We purchased metalized material from Aaronia, a German firm. I found a sewing pattern for a hoody and pair of pants that seemed appropriate and hired a local seamstress to create an outfit for me. As the material is very transparent, I had the outfit made large as I knew it would need to go over my everyday outerwear: pants and blouse. I supplied the seamstress with a cute hat, which she lined and attached long veils all around. I now have full head/face protection and my body is fully covered. This makes a huge difference with the amount of time I can spend in an EMF*d up area. Aaronia material is lighter, softer and more transparent than other material we have experienced, but anything that covers one's whole head tends to be rather confining. The Aaronia material has 50db attenuation.
www.aaronia.com

In experimenting, I found that it is best not to have the material touch your skin. I have airspace between myself and the material by way of the brim of a hat or material of underclothing or lining. It would be a good idea to always carry around your protective gear, as you never know if there was an emergency and you found yourself in an area with high EMFs. Even with our special EMF radiation protective window tinting on our vehicle, I find that in some areas I start feeling ill, the meter reads high radiation, and I must don the headgear until out of that particular area.

Owning an EMF shielding outfit means I can see a doctor and be able to comprehend my visit. I can travel in the car without feeling like I have the flu. I can go into a store for short periods without getting ill, but I get a lot of startled looks. Those places where I know that I can't be in safely, I just avoid. I don't enjoy wearing the protective gear as it seems to be upsetting to onlookers. The public seems to be alarmed about my full outfit, and they don't know how to react. It must be in my human nature to care about what others think, but in this instance, I should not. I asked a woman wearing a *hajib* if she is bothered by others reactions to her apparel. She told me that she was not bothered as she had been wearing her hajib in public her whole life. She was so nice and open and said that I, too, would get used to it.

Wearing my EMF protective headgear, I have even been mocked by a disabled woman in a wheelchair. She rolled right up to me and said, "Oh, now they have beekeepers in the store. I don't see any bees," and she laughed! At first, I got teary-eyed and then told myself to buck up, and told her that "not all disabilities put one in a wheelchair." She apologized. I handed her one of the business card-sized information cards I have made with information on EHS. Hopefully I turned the situation into one of learning for both of us.

My latest venture into public had good results. A wonderful woman, Pat, recognized me through the layers of my veil. We spoke a bit about our days together volunteering, and then she told me I looked mysterious and alluring in my new outfit. This positive statement made me think a little longer on why I wear the outfit. I wear my metalized outfit because I love and respect my body. I wear the outfit for myself so I might be well. I wear my metalized outfit to honor who I am and have

All EMF*d Up

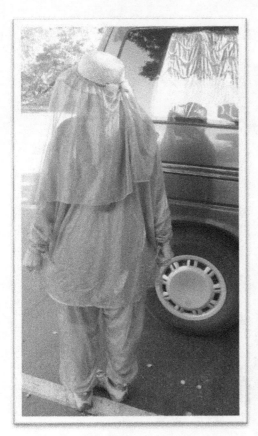

become and feel I am in a contract with my higher self to take care of what I have been gifted. Going forward, I will wear my metalized outfit proudly. Maybe in the near future there will be EMF protective high fashions. Wouldn't that be fun! So, if someone reading this is great in clothing design and fashion, would you please design and sell beautiful EMF-shielded clothing. There are so many people becoming EMF sensitive that business would be booming.

Anne Mills

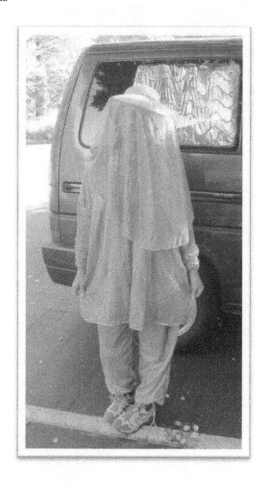

Personal EMF Protection Ideas

There are many online sites that offer items for personal protection from EMF. Many of the items offered smack of fraudulence. These sites give me the sense that someone is trying to make money from a situation where there is not much on the market to help the EHS survivors. I am afraid to admit that I would consider about anything to alleviate this malady. Nonetheless, prior to any purchase it is a good idea to do your own research and read reviews from previous customers. It might be prudent to inquire if others have heard or used a product, perhaps through a chat site. Be aware that what works for one EHS survivor does not always work for everyone, just as not everyone suffers from the same symptoms.

I am in contact with several EHS survivors who use EMF protective shoe inserts and what is called "pocket ground" and "aqua pocket ground," with good results. These can be purchased online at A M Designs Health. Some have reported a lessening of symptoms. I myself have not tried them but they are next on my list, as I have heard good things. It is suggested that with any product held close to the body, to start slowly and build up your use. www.amdesignshealth.com/product-page/earth-pocket-ground .

Following is a link to a government site in which they explain why metallic patches or chips or minerals claimed by sellers to be protective do not seem to make sense and might even be risky. "Shielding Methods and products against man made Electromagnetic Fields: Protection versus Risk" www.ncbi.nlm.nih.gov/pubmed/30831365

There are many crystals, pendants, and signal-blocking phone buttons that come up for sale online for the purpose of EMF shielding. I do not believe any of them work. Some online sites claim copper rods, harmonizers, balancers or neutralizers ward off EMF, and I don't believe they offer anything substantial to those of us with EHS. They all state they're the perfect cure; their advertising seems to solve all the problems that no one else has a solution. I would like to believe that there is a magic pill or a special amulet. The EHS market seems to be ripe for exploiting, so make sure your purchase is returnable. EHS survivors seemingly only have ourselves to rely on, to come to a conclusion about what might help and what doesn't. I have no idea if a product only works for me or it would help someone else. Some items offered for sale, I am sure, are placebo effect, but if it makes you feel better, yay. I tend to be so critical, but still want anything to work, so I tend to try something just in case it is magic. I haven't found it yet.

    After we moved back to the states, I realized that there was no one to turn to for help with the increasing after-effects of my EMF poisoning. There seems to be no scientific or medical research being done in the U.S. for a cure for EHS. I think I've mentioned that the physicians in Europe told me that there was not a cure or reversal for radiation poisoning. As most doctors in the United States are not trained in environmental poisonings, who do we turn to for answers in better health and wellbeing? Eric and I have had several calls from those who believe they have EHS, asking what they should do for themselves. This is a difficult thing to answer, as everyone's EHS and symptoms are special. I can only tell them what we have tried and what worked for us, but that doesn't mean everyone should try things I've tried, or that they would work. The only way I know to feel better, is avoidance of EMF radiation. My doctors in Europe have told me this same thing. The only way to be well is to avoid the source of radiation.

    Eric and I have done our fair share of testing products that might help ease the symptoms of EHS. We tested different Faraday cages and radiation meters, to see which ones worked best for our application and pocketbook. We used our meter to test which window shielding and protective clothing worked best. I have experimented with supplements from organic suppliers. If a supplement is shown to help the brain, I try it. There are medallions and lockets for sale on the market that I have tried. They did not help me. I have purchased Shungite crystals, though I can't say I noticed a difference in using them. Neither Amazonite crystals nor pink salt candle holders worked, in my instance, to help alleviate EMF from my computer screen. A couple of people have reported help from magnets but I don't like the way they feel.

So, I admit that I am an optimist, or desperado, that does try to find something to help my EHS symptoms. I read product reviews and try to speak with others who have also tried a product. Who do we turn to when we need help with health, when there are no experiments and research in the U.S. outside of those paid for by industry? Scrutinize all research that says there is no ill health effects from EMF, as there is a good chance they are paid for by industry. The telecom industry only invests in and publishes those research outcomes that prove no health risk from electromagnetic field radiation.

EHS support group: www.es-forum.com
                     www.wearetheevidence.org

Again, please note: These are things I have tried for my own situation. In no way should you risk your health or well-being on the advice of something I tried, as every situation is different. Please research prudently and come to your own conclusions. Please consult your physician before experimenting with supplements, especially if you are taking other drugs.

Anne Mills

Traveling Safely with EHS

      Traveling safely with EHS has become more difficult in the last several years due to proliferation of EMF sources. As with most people, our main mode of transport is a car, which means we utilize the freeways to a large extent. The main problem is that these freeways are lined with cell phone towers emitting radiation and our destination is usually All EMF*d Up also. To protect ourselves when traveling, we always look up our destination address on www.AntennaSearch.com. This tells us how far from our destination the offending cell tower and antenna are located. An antenna search shows the cell towers and antennae within a four-mile radius of the address entered. Recently we have found cases where Antenna Search does not list all towers or antenna. This may be due to the fact that the companies are not required to register and possibly the industry doesn't want you to know about all erected towers.
      I also have to be cognizant of closer sources of radiation, like WiFi. Since most people look for broadband, it is a rare hotel, hostel, or BnB that doesn't advertise free WiFi. We do call and ask if they can unplug the WiFi router, but most lodging management is unwilling or unable to do so. We also need to be careful of the traveler in the adjoining room that might have a laptop or notebook with a hot spot. This is difficult to guard against. We also unplug any wireless appliances we find in the room. Remember, also, that free WiFi is the opposite of WiFi-free.
      Plane travel was a necessity when living in Germany, but plane travel had become painful. On our final flight moving from Germany back to California, as we were about to land I had a terrible experience. I developed a pain in my head that entailed terrible head pressure giving way to blurry vision. Nothing I did helped alleviate the pain and I almost blacked out. We attribute this to passengers turning their cell phones on before we landed.

This was in 2009, and is the last time I traveled by air. It was also before we owned a radiation meter or any personal EMF protective gear. I would suggest if you have protective head shielding, put it on well before landing. Eric has flown in the meantime and the EMF radiation reading both on the plane and in the airport pegged the meter.

I was hoping train travel might be a safe venue, and made inquiries at Amtrak and American-by-Rail, but they all seem to have WiFi. A downside of train travel would be other travelers and their wireless devices. Outside of asking them to turn off their phones, I figured this mode of transport is too restrictive for my well-being. The cruise ships have WiFi for all passengers. I will continue to search for a safe form of travel.

Window Tinting

When driving, we found that before we reached our destination, I was ill from all the antenna that line the highway. Our meters have shown that the cell phone antenna along freeways spew high levels of EMFs. I always wear my EMF protective headgear in the vehicle, but sometimes this gets stifling and uncomfortable to wear for many hours at a time.

Eric found a window tinting that is made in Canada for the CIA and State Department for anti-eavesdropping. He purchased this film from Safe Living Technologies Inc. It is referred to as "Signal Protect Clear". (www.slt.co/Products) It is only slightly tinted and presents no problem for night driving and no issue with law enforcement. It's important to have an experienced installer as this material is not stretchy like auto glass tinting, as it is made for buildings (flat glass). Apparently, the early auto glass tinting was not so stretchy and this is where the experience is helpful. (The owner of the window tinting firm installed ours.) Please note that initially there will be large bubbling of water between the film and the glass, which only slowly subsides. It would be advantageous to wait until the warmer months of the year to do this project. In areas of hot weather, I would expect it to dry out much quicker, perhaps over a couple of days. Before the bubbles disappear, you would not want to drive at night as the bubbles are very distracting. Once the bubbles clear, it is very transparent. (also see the Protective Shelters chapter) We are very careful how we clean the inside surfaces, so as not to scratch the window film. On our vehicle, all the glass on windows that open are covered on the inside up to the very edge of the window. For the fixed glass, they installed it as close to the rubber seals as possible. A hole was cut out of the tinting on the front window where the rear-view mirror is attached. With no other shielding, the reduction in cabin was ~ 98.9%, as measured by Eric Windheim, a certified building biologist in our area specializing in EMF solutions. www.windheimemfsolutions.com.

Important Note: Please do not use your cell phone in your vehicle. If you use your cell phone in your vehicle, you are unwittingly intensifying your EMF exposure. Your auto is metal and acts like a Faraday cage, similar to the microwave oven enclosure that tries to keep EMFs inside of itself. This makes it more difficult for your phone to talk to the cell tower. When this happens, your phone amps up, "talks louder" to the cell tower, and in doing this puts up to ten times more radiation into the cabin. The user's manuals for vehicles sold in Europe actually state the dangers and warn of using a cell phone without an external antenna.

Suggestions for Travel:
- Always bring your radiation meter.
- Have your EMF protective clothing and/or EMF protective sleeping bag close at hand.
- Pack some of your own food in case you are unable to find restaurants free of radiation or get food ordered to go.

- We always pack our Stetzer filters, as it really quiets the whole room.
- Make sure you have a plan B.

Anne Mills

Healing and Recovery from an EMF poisoning
Lessons Learned

Electromagnetic field Radiation compromises your immune system, making the body unable to protect itself and repair. Upon issuing my diagnosis of Electromagnetic Hypersensitivity, my physician in Germany, Dr. Eger, explained that due to the excessive exposure, my body had become unable to protect itself and repair. He explained that my blood test showed that my red blood cell count had collapsed and my vitamin D count was alarmingly low. EMF radiation is dangerous to our wellbeing as a whole, but the two organs that are most vulnerable are the heart and the brain. It is well documented that these fields can compromise the blood brain barrier, a filter that blocks toxins from entering the brain. The blood brain barrier prevents damage to the central nervous system. Wireless radiation can cause blood brain barrier leakage. EHS (electromagnetic sensitivity) was a life changing and very scary edict. There are thousands of peer-reviewed scientific studies showing a myriad of damaging effects EMFs can cause. My favorite sites are www.EHTrust.org and www.MDsafetech.org.

Having been grossly poisoned by EMFs, I am so grateful to my physicians in Germany for their concern and support. These are the recommendations they gave me as well as some that I have learned on my own:

1. Get a Good Night's Sleep

My physician told me it was imperative to get a good nights' sleep, as this is when your body does much of its healing. Radiation impairs your body's ability to produce melatonin, a natural sleep hormone and a powerful antioxidant. Melatonin can reverse oxidative stress that results from radiation. Insomnia is a symptom of EHS. I was first prescribed Baldrian, an herbal sleep aid that is called Valerian here in the United States. This herbal sleep aid did not seem to help after about a week, so Dr. Eger prescribed melatonin in the form of a natural supplement. Melatonin worked well in helping me get to and stay asleep and did not produce any ill effects in the morning. As I was still feeling the physical effects of the massive EMF radiation poisoning, the only thing that helped me accomplish deep sleep was the Faraday cage that Eric built. (see chapter on Protective Shelters, Faraday cage.) The Faraday cage was the best gift Eric ever made for me as it screened out the EMF. My doctor also suggested that I get sunlight daily, as this not only offers Vitamin D naturally, but helps the body produce its own melatonin.

It is crucial to minimize the EMF in your sleeping area. Dr. Heinlein at the Medical University at Coberg stated that it is most important to eliminate sources of radiation during REM sleep. There should be no wireless devices in or around the bedroom. I suggest that prior to going to bed you turn off all wireless devices and refrain from using cell phones/laptops, as the blue light triggers melatonin suppression. I personally turn off all electrical devices in the bedroom and switch off all the rooms' power breakers. If you have EHS symptoms after going to bed and your EMF meter shows EMF sources, you might need a Faraday shelter.

2. Eat Healthy, Stay Hydrated

It's extremely important to eat healthy by reducing your intake of sugar and non-organic foods, trying to eat nutritionally and organically. I credit my healing in part to eating lots of organic greens and vegetables. I believe a healthy gut is imperative to recovery from any illness, EHS included. I always include probiotics in my supplements. A dietician suggested I limit my dairy to aged cheese and organic butter. Since surviving breast cancer in 2012, I've craved cilantro and eat it in huge amounts; maybe half a cup on a dinner salad. I also grow and eat the herb purslane, known as a weed by many, on the suggestion of an organic farmer in our area. He went as far as delivering it to my house when I was too ill with cancer to go to the local farmers market. He told me it is very high in Omega 3. Purslane is difficult to find, but very easy to grow. Because blueberries are good for brain health, I now grow blueberries in my garden.

Stay Hydrated: Avoid getting dehydrated. Drink pure water, preferably not from plastic containers. Green tea is good for brain health. On occasion, I have experienced vertigo after extreme exercise and have found that liquid with electrolytes have helped much more than plain water. I now carry half water, half coconut water when exercising as coconut water is high in natural electrolytes. (Also, be aware that as we age our ability to sense dehydration diminishes.)

3. Exercise, Meditation and Grounding:

Exercise boosts your immune system, oxygenates the blood, helps to fight cancers and slows the aging process. Another big benefit of exercise is how it helps fight depression.

Meditation lessens anxiety, depression, and pain. It also, among other benefits, improves sleep and reduces stress.

Grounding. I always ground myself prior to meditating. When I ground, I feel as if I'm sloughing off unwanted effects of EMF energy, like a big sigh of relief. I have recently learned that grounding, or earthing, is not safe everywhere, as the American utility companies don't use a neutral lead back to their power stations, as they do in Europe. In the United States, the utility companies rely on the earth to connect current, which can make the earth extremely electrified along this return path. Now I'm more aware of where I am grounding and make sure I am in an isolated area.

https://articles.mercola.com/sites/articles/archive/2018/01/20/grounding-benefits.aspx

4. Fasting

I believe that fasting is beneficial, and I fast several days a week by eating a late breakfast (11:00 AM) and an early dinner (5:00 PM) with nothing after dinner. I read that apple cider vinegar taken daily is good for you. Every day I down a tablespoon with an equal amount of water in a shot glass, followed by a large glass of water as a chaser.

5. Supplements

I know that it is important to eat your vitamins in the form of greens, but because I can't always eat enough of the good stuff to equal what is recommended, I take supplements. In Germany, I was given a prescription for large amounts of zinc to help boost my immune system. I was told to drink electrolytes in the form of a type of Gatorade they had available there. Electrolytes can be purchased in tablets, liquid drops, and powders. I was also told to take large amounts of omega-3s, magnesium, and vitamin D, which helps your body absorb magnesium. I enjoy organic Tulsi Holy Basil tea and believe it helps strengthen my immune system. (Contact your physician before you take any supplements to make sure they won't conflict with medications you're taking.)

<u>Turmeric</u>: I take turmeric for brain health, as it's known to be both an anti-inflammatory and anti-oxidant as well as having microbial and anti-cancer properties. Among many other benefits, turmeric protects your body against radiation-induced damage and heavy metal toxicity and is capable of crossing your blood-brain barrier, acting as a possible neuro-protective agent for neurological disorders such as Parkinson's and Alzheimer's diseases. (Caution: Not everyone should take turmeric, as it is a blood thinner and could cause liver problems.)

<u>Magnesium</u>: The physicians in Germany suggested I take magnesium. I took it at night as it upset my stomach during the day. Upon moving back to the United States, I found

magnesium l-threonate didn't upset my stomach. Per studies by Dr. Martin Pall, EMFs affect one's voltage-gated calcium channels, and magnesium acts as a natural calcium-channel blocker, lowering the effects of EMFs. I consider magnesium and vitamin D to be the two most important supplements I take.

<u>Vitamin D3</u>. When we moved back to California, my physician found that my vitamin D blood levels were extremely low and prescribed 50,000 iu (International Units) every three days. Since then, I've taken between 5,000 and 10,000 iu daily, depending on how much sun I'm able to enjoy. Vitamin D not only helps with magnesium absorption but acts as an antidepressant. I try to get a yearly blood test that includes vitamin D counts.

<u>Omega 3s</u>: Omega-3 fatty acids are imperative for brain health; they help preserve the integrity of your blood-brain barrier. I get my omega-3 by taking krill oil capsules. My doctor suggested I start adding an omega-3 count to my blood test.

<u>Astaxanthin</u>: Per the National Institute of Health, astaxanthin supplements were "shown to protect neurons in experimental models of acute injuries, chronic neurode-generative disorders, and neurological diseases and was proposed as a beneficial strategy to treat neurological diseases. Astaxanthin chelates several metal ions, and has anti-inflammatory properties. Astaxanthin crosses the blood brain barrier, allowing free access to the central nervous system."

<u>Vitamin B and liposomal Vit.C.</u> I take an array of these supplements.

<u>Vit. K2.</u> (for bone health) Per Dr. Andrew Weil: Vitamin K is necessary for normal blood clotting, and it regulates calcium in the body, keeping it in the bones and out of the arteries. Adequate vitamin K intake also appears to reduce the risks of both heart disease and cancer. **Through my reading and also speaking with a dietician, I learned that it is best if you eat your calcium.** Sources of high calcium foods include tofu, milk, yogurt, cheese, leafy greens, beans, clams, okra, trout, and

acorn squash and sardines. (Vitamin K should not be taken by anyone taking anticoagulant medications.)

NRF2 Renew: Dr. Martin Pall suggested that I take NRF2, a natural supplement that, among other functions, lowers inflammation, improves mitochondrial function, and helps the body detoxify from everyday toxins and EMFs. I purchase the NRF2 supplement through Allergy Research Group. I feel it helps lessen the affects I would feel from exposure to EMF. Eating vegetables, especially from the cruciferous/cabbage family, as well as high intensity exercise and intermittent fasting also help increase NRF2 naturally.

(Please check with your physician to make sure that the supplements you choose do not negatively react with your prescriptions.)

6. Remove Metal Dental Fillings

While still in Germany and under the direction of my doctors, I had a dentist remove metal fillings in my teeth. I still had one metal filling left in my mouth when we moved back to California, and was told by the dentist that removed it, that it was half silver and half gold, like a little battery.

EMF Detox

Eric and I were fortunate to have German physicians who knew about EMFs and their ill effects. What we didn't realize was that what I did to help myself recover and heal from my poisoning event was called "detox.: In reading up on what is involved in detox for EMFs, it reads pretty much as I've listed above:

1. Avoid all EMFs – I just stopped cold turkey. Not as easy for everyone.
2. Protect against EMFs by knowing their sources (Get a radiation meter)

3. Eat well, go organic, drink lots of pure water, (Coconut water has needed electrolytes)
Some foods that naturally detox your body: asparagus, avocados, broccoli, cilantro, garlic, ginger, kelp and tomatoes.
4. Exercise to oxygenate your blood and activate NRF2, which boosts your brain health.
5. Find a safe EMF-free place to sleep, the time when your body does most of it's healing.
6. Grounding/earthing are important ways to slough off unwanted energy.
7. Taking beneficial supplements like NRF2 Renew helps with detox, as does magnesium; they both help your body heal.
8. Try salt and soda tub soaks. I've read that some EHS sufferers submerge themselves in warm baths of half ionized salt, half baking soda. I haven't done this, as I don't have a bath tub.

Directions for a Salt and Soda Soak:
    https://branchbasics.com/blog/salt-and-soda-soak-a-radiation-detox-bath/
I've also heard that clay or mud baths are beneficial for radiation detox. I haven't used this treatment, but I'm willing to try it if I can find a spa or treatment facility that doesn't emit radiation with their wireless music and communication devices while I try to purge radiation.

<u>Try Chelation Therapy or Not</u>: I used to be able to shop or meet friends in a pub or even sit out at the pier with friends to watch the surfers ride the waves and the fishermen bring in their boats. I am no longer able to do those things. I don't know if I'm becoming more sensitive, but I *do* know there are more and more EMFs in our environment, as our meters tell us the readings are huge. In wondering if I had become more sensitive to EMFs, I started thinking about how I've been told that metal acts like an antenna. I had already had all my metal fillings removed years ago, but thought it might be prudent to find other ways to help

myself. This year I purchased plastic eyeglasses. I've also stopped wearing my large metal dangly earrings. So what about my internal metals? I had chemo to treat my breast cancer in 2011 and heard that chemo uses heavy metals. Are those metals still in my body? I need to find out about chelation therapy and what that involves. Do I need to test for which metals or does chelation therapy remove them all? Maybe if there are no metals present in my body I will be less sensitive. I've spoken to a couple EHS (electromagnetic sensitive) survivors who have tried this, and it is time to take it on myself. When I told my physician my plan, I was advised that in my case I first needed a blood test for metal toxicity, which I have not done yet

EMFs in Pregnancy and with Young Children

I was lucky that I wasn't pregnant during the introduction of wireless devices and the subsequent huge explosion of microwave radiation. For those pregnant women who are aware of their surroundings, our new EMF'd up environment makes it a particularly challenging time. There is not only a growing list of studies that show an increase in miscarriages, but studies showing negative effects on fetus and children exposed to EMF in utero; lower memory, increased hyperactivity, asthma, obesity in offspring, to name a few. There are also studies showing increase in autism-like symptoms in children that have now been linked to the presence of EMFs. www.ehtrust.org

A Yale study found cell phone radiation exposure caused mice exposed prenatally to have "ADHD-like" symptoms of hyperactivity and poor memory. In response to this growing body of research, obstetricians, medical doctors, and public health educators have signed onto a major initiative called The Baby Safe Project, which recommends that pregnant women reduce wireless exposure to protect their unborn babies' developing brains. www.babysafeproject.org

I do not have experience with trying to raise a child in an EMF*d up environment. When our son was growing up, I did not have awareness and knowledge of wireless radiation. I have only read of and have heartfelt sadness for those families who have had to deal with negative health impacts on their children due to EMF. I can only offer a few online sites as a help.

"Health effects of non ionizing radiation on children" Toril Jelter, Pediatrician (YouTube)

For information on the relationship between autism and EMFs
https://www.bioinitiative.org/report/wp-content/uploads/pdfs/sec20/2012_Findings_in_Autism.pdf

Abstract
Mobile phones and other wireless devices that produce electromagnetic fields (EMF) and pulsed radiofrequency radiation (RFR) are widely documented to cause potentially harmful health impacts that can be detrimental to young people. New epigenetic studies are profiled in this review to account for some neurodevelopmental and neurobehavioral changes due to exposure to wireless technologies. Symptoms of retarded memory, learning, cognition, attention, and behavioral problems have been reported in numerous studies and are similarly manifested in autism and attention deficit hyperactivity disorders, as a result of EMF and RFR exposures where both epigenetic drivers and genetic (DNA) damage are likely contributors. Technology benefits can be realized by adopting wired devices for education to avoid health risk and promote academic achievement. © 2017 The Authors. Child Development © 2017 Society for Research in Child Development, Inc.
https://www.ncbi.nlm.nih.gov/pubmed/28504324

Camilla Rees – Screen Time in Schools –Biological Effects of Electromagnetic Radiation
https://www.youtube.com/watch?v=JS8BnEYaVcI

http://www.clearlightventures.com/blog/2015/9/11/the-emerging-link-between-wireless-and-autism

http://naturalhealthforlife.com/autism/research-dangers-emfs-autism

For information on the links between miscarriages and EMFs
https://www.emfacts.com/2018/01/miscarriage-risks-linked-to-electromagnetic-field-exposure-power-frequency-elf-magnetic-fields/

If you've been able to find products or professionals that have helped alleviate your symptoms of EHS and help you lead a normal and social life, please share with other EHS survivors. There is a definite lack of independent studies in the area of our healing, so we have to rely on eachother. Recovery from EHS has to be a concerted effort.

Heartfelt wishes in your search for better health. Anne

Diagnosis, Disability and ADA

Diagnosis

As a short recap from the beginning journal section of the book, I was poisoned, physically injured, with electromagnetic field radiation (EMF) while we lived in a small town in Germany. The radiation strength and frequency readings from a cell phone tower were measured at gross and illegally high levels. The readings went to the Germany court system. I went to doctors as an ill and very scared victim. My husband, Eric, and I spent over two hours on our initial visit with Dr. Horst Eger, as he took notes on my health history and that of my family. He questioned us about our habits and living environment. Dr. Eger wrote prescriptions for blood testing, neurological tests, gynecology tests, and made an appointment for us with an internist. He ordered tests to rule out all other causes. Dr. Eger gave me a diagnosis of Electromagnetic Hypersensitivity (EHS) in May of 2007. He explained this malady and how this would affect me for the rest of my life. He warned me of lingering ill effects and possible cancers in the plural. He also gave suggestions that would assist in my healing and wrote prescriptions to that end. Dr. Eger proceeded to call me every week to check on my rehabilitation. This is an example of a great physician.

If you are a reader who believes you have EHS, first do all you can to mitigate the EMF that are negatively impacting your health. Take the necessary steps to alleviate EMF from your home/work space: shielding window tint, shielding wall paper or paint, aluminum window screens, etc. (see chapters on Protective Shelters and Personal Protection.) It would be a good idea to document EMF readings, and to do this you need to purchase a good meter, learn how to use it, and take a video or pictures of the readings in each of the rooms of your home. You could also hire a building biologist and I believe it is part of their service that they provide a written radiation reading review of your home. Then take new video or pictures of the now-lower EMF in your living/work space. Keep lists, receipts, records of monies spent in your efforts to a healthier lifestyle. Keep a journal and note if your symptoms have improved. Improvement might take a couple months. The key is to document everything.

If those actions help your health, then you are already into establishing proof of your EHS. Find a doctor that is open-minded. Print out peer-reviewed scientific medical research that supports your belief and present them to the doctor. There are many studies on EHS to be found on www.mdsafetech.org or www.ehtrust.org. Show your physician how you were able to change your environment and how those changes affected your health for the better. Why do you think you got EHS? Did you keep a timeline/diary of symptoms? Does your work record show a problem with health issues? I also had to produce letters of "attest," as they are called in Europe, from my doctors who gave me the diagnosis in Germany. These "attest" documents explain my health prior to illness, the new diagnosis, why, and when. It would be a good idea to show your physician the symptoms you have documented. I gave Dr. Eger my diary observations.

A letter of diagnosis should state that you, the patient, have Electromagnetic Sensitivity (EMS as known in the U.S). It should make clear that being in proximity to electromagnetic fields exacerbates your symptoms. Your physician could go on to say that it is imperative that you, for instance, not have a smart meter, or work in a situation that does not have wireless router or wireless devices in the vicinity, or that purchase and application of special window tinting is advised. My letters of diagnosis do not have my symptoms. The following is a link to a United Kingdom EHS site that has sample letters of diagnosis under resources: www.es-uk.info

Eric and I consider ourselves lucky that in Germany we were able to find such a renowned doctor who knew the cause of

EHS, the symptoms, and how to help me recover. Here in the United States, few of the physicians seem to be trained in environmental illnesses. I have heard of physicians in the United States being ostracized for their belief of EHS by their fellow peers. So how does one get a diagnosis for EHS when physicians in the U.S. are not trained in EMF poisoning? You could talk to others who have a diagnosis and get the name of their physician. I believe there is an effort to make a blood test that shows EHS. I have seen brain CT scans that show the difference between those brains that have been affected by EMF versus those brains that have not. I do not know if at this time they are using this method for diagnosis, but a knowledgeable physician might know.

This article, by Prof. Dominique Belpomme, a leading clinical researcher, states that there are diagnostic tests, and that EHS can be: "routinely diagnosed by commercially available simple biological tests... The disorder involves inflammation-related hyper-histaminemia, oxidative stress, autoimmune response, capsulothalamic hyperfusion and BBB [blood brain barrier] opening, and a deficit in melatonin metabolic..." http://www.ncbi.nlm.nih.gov/pubmed/26613326.

An article that would be smart to share with your doctor is the scientific review from "EUROPAEM EMF Guideline 2016, for the prevention, diagnosis, and treatment of EMF-related health problems and illnesses" Full text: https://www.ncbi.nlm.nih.gov/pubmed/27454111

It is imperative that we have physicians in the United States acquire training in environmental illness and the hazardous effects of EMF. I believe that there is not a doctor in the U.S. who has a patient that has not come in contact with EMF, not even the Amish. With ever mounting evidence that EMF cause a myriad of diseases; we need to push for physician training.

Social Security Disability Insurance – SSDI

As I could no longer work due to my Electromagnetic Sensitivity (EHS) (or Radiation Sickness), in 2010 I decided that it would be prudent to apply for disability. I considered my EHS a disability, as I can no longer hold a job. I had worked for well over twenty years in the administrative assistant field. How would I be able to accomplish this now? Where would I get gainful employment? Was there an office that was not by any cell tower or antenna and could that office assure me that they or a neighboring office did not utilize wireless equipment? Was there an office I could work in that as clients enter I could demand that they turn off their cell phones and wireless devices?

I was quick to realize that this was not a normal disability case, as my lawyer had no experience in EMF poisoning. I had to supply the lawyer with information and scientific/medical peer reviewed research papers regarding EHS. Every time I found new research, I sent it to the lawyer. I also presented to him all the measured radiation readings that were taken in Germany at the time of the poisoning. I presented my written diagnosis from physicians and all communications from the German and American Consulate. I submitted all information I had to the lawyer, and prayed.

To the courts, I showed proof of years of contributing to Social Security. I had many letters from people witnessing my symptoms of EHS. We showed myriads of receipts on our attempts to mitigate EMF intrusion for health sake by way of protective clothing and monies spent on shielding material for housing. We gave evidence of how EHS had changed our lifestyle, our move to a rural area due to EMF, and how we had to live apart to continue his employment.

My physician in Germany, Dr. Eger, had worked for many years in studies proving that EMFs have been linked to ill health and cancers. He also has written my poisoning case up in several medical journals. I was able to obtain diagnosis letters from several doctors here in California. Applying for disability means not only filling out forms but a myriad of visits to court-appointed doctors and psychologists. All of this took lots of time and lots of travel.

In a very rare verdict, with the help from my physician Dr. Eger; my wonderful lawyer, since retired; his staff, occupational experts, my brave husband, and after two years and one appeal, I was awarded *full permanent* SSI disability based on Electromagnetic HyperSensitivity. This was in 2012. Eric and I were aware that this was an unusual case, but not aware that this was anything but a normal judgment. I received disability based on EHS. It was not until after the judgment that we were cautioned not to speak of it to anyone. We were told I was the first in the United States to receive such an award, and we were not sure where the attention would take the ruling. In the following article from Germany, I am referred to as a man:

"When a US American patient moved to Bavaria in 2006 and he was sensitized by nocturnal High Frequency radiation, he had to move away in 2007, but although he improved he was unable to work subsequently because of the ever higher environmental exposures. The court acknowledged his ES in 2012 and he was granted a pension back-dated to 2008". (Eger H. "Causal Legally Recognized Proof of the Damage Potential of Technical Highfrequency Fields – A Case Report" Umwelt-medizin-gesellschaft, 2014)

I understand that many have attempted to gain disability for EHS, but instead had to label their illness either Multiple Sclerosis, Multiple Chemical Sensitivity (MCS), or other autoimmune diseases. I knew of only one other person who was granted disability for EHS, and his was derived from an experienced occupational hazard from his past employment. It's always such a shock when the papers reveal that a woman got temporary disability for EHS in France, or a man in Australia got disability for three years. I believe that, like me, there must be those with disability related to EHS that are hesitant to say anything and have been warned to keep quiet.

Americans with Disability Act – ADA

The Americans with Disabilities Act (ADA) became law in 1990. The ADA is a civil rights law that prohibits discrimination against individuals with disabilities in all areas of public life, including jobs, schools, transportation, and all public and private places that are open to the general public. The purpose of the law is to make sure that people with disabilities have the same civil rights, protections and opportunities as everyone else, similar to those provided to individuals on the basis of race, color, sex, national origin, age, and religion.
"It guarantees equal opportunity for individuals with disabilities in public accommodations, employment, transportation, state and local government services, and telecommunications."
www.adata.org/learn-about-ada

Americans with Disability Act is centered on what one is unable to accomplish due to a disability. Due to my EMF poisoning I cannot do my own shopping and I cannot maintain a socially active lifestyle anymore. I would like to remain a contributing member of society. I know that we pay, as citizens, for the library that I can no longer enjoy, due to their high levels of EMF. I can no longer go to a movie, concert, restaurants, or a nice pub. I cannot enter a government office; they are all EMF*d up. How am I going to go to the DMV? Due to my EHS, I can't take public transportation because all buses now have WiFi, as do planes and trains. There is no school/public education facility that has an area free of EMF radiation. Hospitals, emergency rooms, clinics all have exorbitant EMF radiation. I do not know how the U.S. is going to handle the new disability of EHS. Some of the highest levels of radiation shown by our meters are at the physician's office. How are these public places of business going to establish "safe" areas for the new disability? At the very least, there should be "White Zones," zones where there is no detectible EMF, in all medical establishments. (see chapter on White Zones.)

In order to establish claims under the Federal Americans with Disabilities Act, (ADA), the plaintiff must establish that he was disabled within the meaning of the ADA. The ADA defines a "disability" as: 1) a physical or mental impairment that substantially limits one or more major life activities; 2) a record of such impairment; or 3) an individual that is regarded as having such an impairment. The referred to "one or more major life activities" include caring for oneself, sleeping, learning, and concentrating. There is currently no code in the ADA book for EHS.

I know that the ADA has not caught up with the real-world applications of technology in regards to making sure public buildings are in compliance and made accessible to those with EHS. Noted below is an excerpt from IEQ: Indoor Environmental Quality, a project of the National Institute of Building Sciences (NIBS) with funding support from the Architectural and Transportation Barriers Compliance Board (Access Board). They have given recommendations for ADA access for those with EHS and MCS starting on page 48.

> "Conditions of Use The Cleaner Air Symbol may be posted to identify the room and path of travel if there is verification that the room, facility, and path of travel to the room meet all of the Cleaner Air Requirements as indicated below: • No Smoking • Fragrance-Free • Pesticide-Free (Indoors and Outdoors) • Least Toxic/Risk Cleaning Products • No Recent Construction or Remodeling Including Carpet Installation • Cell phones turned off • Ability to turn off or unplug computers and other electrical equipment by occupant or staff • Ability to turn off fluorescent lighting by occupant or staff • Ability to adjust temperature and air flow by occupant or staff, or the availability of operable window(s)"

https://web.archive.org/web/20060714175343/ieq.nibs.org/ieq_project.pdf

As noted by Smart Meter Harm (www.smartmeterharm.org),"After acknowledging electromagnetic sensitivity (EMS) in 2002, the U.S. Access Board contracted with the National Institute of Building Sciences (NIBS) to develop an Indoor Environmental Quality project, the first step in the Access Board's 'action plan to reduce the level of chemicals and electromagnetic fields in the built environment' for the EMF-disabled and those disabled by multiple chemical sensitivities. In 2005, NIBS released a 97-page Indoor Environmental Quality report, containing extensive recommendations and resources. The report and its sections are on the Access Board's website here:" www.access-board.gov/research/completed-research/indoor-environmental-quality

The U.S. Access Board has taken the commentary very seriously and acted upon it. As stated in the *Background for its Final Rule Americans with Disabilities Act (ADA) Accessibility Guidelines for Buildings and Facilities; Recreation Facilities* that was published in September 2002, the Board recognizes that multiple chemical sensitivities and electromagnetic sensitivities may be considered disabilities under the ADA if they so severely impair the neurological, respiratory or other functions of an individual that it substantially limits one or more of the individual's major life activities. The Access Board plans to closely examine the needs of this population, and undertake activities that address accessibility issues for these individuals." www.access-board.gov/research/completed-research/indoor-environmental-quality

Following its recognition of electrosensitivity and its declaration of commitment to attend to the needs of the

electromagnetic sensitive, the Access Board contracted the National Institute of Building Sciences (NIBS) to examine how to accommodate the needs of the electro sensitive in federally funded buildings. In 2005 the NIBS issued a report. The link for the report:
http://web.archive.org/web/20060714175343/ieq.nibs.org/ieq_project.pdf

For questions/comments/complaints regarding EHS compliancy:
https://www.epa.gov/aboutepa/about-office-air-and-radiation-oar#oria

Until we have physicians that can diagnose EHS, and until EHS is considered a real disability by ADA, there will be few concessions made for our living a more normal life. It took decades for enough pressure to be exerted on cities to tear out their sidewalks and make ramps for wheelchairs. How long will it take, how many people will have to be EHS disabled, before we have white zones in a doctor's office or a safe environment for surgery?

I do not see where ADA has helped in my quest to live a more normal life. This is not going to change in the current climate of industry holding rein over government by the people, for the people, unless the people make known that they are not happy and they want change. Your vote counts. Your money talks. Make purchases wisely. Write to your elected officials.

It is a sad day when the only thing that wakes up industry to the harm they are causing humans and environment, is when it hits their bottom line in the form of lawsuits. I believe the day will soon come. The wireless industries know of the dangers of EMF, as do their investors. Lloyd's of London is one of the largest insurance underwriters in the world. Attached is a recent renewal policy which, as of Feb. 7, 2015, excludes any coverage associated with exposure to non-ionizing radiation. In response to clarification, this response was received on Feb. 18,

2015 from CFC Underwriting LTD, London, UK agent for Lloyd's:
> "The Electromagnetic Fields Exclusion (Exclusion 32) is a General Insurance Exclusion and is applied across the market as standard. The purpose of the exclusion is to exclude cover for illnesses caused by continuous long-term non-ionizing radiation exposure i.e. through mobile phone usage."

This means that insurance companies have chosen not to insure wireless industry for damage from emitted radiation, and wireless industry has notified their shareholders of this fact, but the warnings have been held back from consumers. Following is an excerpt from Complete Markets insurance website regarding lack of coverage for lawsuits based on electromagnetic fields:
> "Electromagnetic field exclusions" are clear and common in most insurance companies. It is applied as a market standard. This exclusion serves to exclude cover for illnesses caused by long-term EMF (non-ionizing radiation) exposure. For EMF liability insurance cover you have to purchase additional "Pollution Liability" coverage. EMF liability insurance covers claims brought by third parties for body injuries and property claims by third parties. This policy does not pay for damage caused by artificially generated electromagnetic, magnetic and electrical energy that damages, disrupts or interferes with any device, appliance, system, electronic wire or network utilizing satellite or cellular technology.

www.completemarkets.com/Electromagnetic-Fields-Utilities-Liability-Insurance

"Don't be afraid to take big steps. You can't cross a chasm in two small jumps."

David Lloyd George (1863-1945)

Anne Mills

Fight or Flight

I had never experienced "fight or flight" until I became an EHS sufferer. I am a normally quiet and congenial person that since becoming sensitive to wireless radiation, has found myself either verbally agitated or walking away from seemingly normal or pleasant situations. My callous actions leave me embarrassed and puzzled as to why. I then realized that "fight or flight" only introduces itself to me in areas with high EMF. This is not a symptom that forewarns with confusion or headaches, but the feeling is suddenly there. I have no say in how the situation or "fight or flight" response comes about; I just react. I am not even cognizant that I am in a situation I don't know how to handle. I am in an all EMF*d up environment that shadows a situation and I either leave or get mad for seemingly no reason.

In one incident, I was visiting with a friend in a small local town that I know has large amounts of EMFs but willfully ignored that fact. Lena and I were just standing outside in front of quaint storefronts, talking. The next thing I know, I realize that Lena was waiting for an answer and I had no idea what she said. She continued to speak but I could not understand a single word, as if she spoke a different language. I suddenly had heart palpitations, a sense of being overwhelmed, a feeling of fear and confusion. I turned and walked quickly away. This is flight. Not planned, not thought about, just my feet did a one-eighty and walked away. I don't know where I am headed but I am out of a threatening situation and into a different one, as I have no idea where to go. This has happened several times when speaking with physicians. I believe it is due to the high EMF in clinics and hospitals. I find myself grabbing my clothes and purse and leaving. This is scary.

I have met my "fight" response, but I think it rears its head as "pissy." I volunteer for a community center. One day working and quite focused on my goal, I realize that I am feeling hot flashes in a room that is cold. Then I realize that all my teeth hurt and I am becoming nauseated and foggy brained. I have a sudden feeling of excitability and anger about working and being subject to EMF from... it dawns on me... someone's cell phone! I am instantly agitated and verbally upset. The first thing I do is put up my head and look for a cell phone, and when I find it, I loudly blurt out, "turn your phone off or get out!" There is no diplomacy even glimmered. I am in pain, I know why, I need to get rid of the offender, so, "get out."

I am not a mean or undiplomatic person, and really, the only time I am rude is when I am in the pain from EMFs. I have never seen medical research stating that "ill-tempered" was a symptom, but it must be an offshoot of "fight." Seemingly, being nice or realizing who I am speaking to or in what situation does not even enter into the picture. This automatic outburst is like a side dish to "fight or flight," or " pissy." Along with "fight or flight" is a "freeze" response that I have not had issue with. Scott Eberle has written a wonderful and comprehensive article on dealing with "fight or flight" and other EHS symptoms. Search *An Underworld Journey, Learning to Cope With Electromagnetic Hypersensitivity*, by Scott Eberle.

I have read that "fight or flight" is known as a stress response; that EMF can trigger your brain to think there is danger but your brain can't perceive if this danger is real or not. This leads to stress and this in turn can lead to your body making adrenalin and stress hormones, which then can lower immune system, possibly leading to autoimmune disorders, affect blood pressure, and lead to heart disease or strokes. This site has in depth information on the brain and "fight or flight." www.drlam.com/blog/how-the-fight-and-flight-response-impacts-the-body/26138

I believe that everyone responds to stress differently, so it is a good idea to understand how you, as an individual, react to stress. Do you freeze or run, get an upset stomach or muscle crams, or get pissy?

Depression

I am not a doctor. I have no training in psychology. I have only been to a counselor once and that was court mandated for disability insurance. Prior to EHS, I had no real knowledge in depression. The experiences I relay are just that; steps I took to make myself feel better. If you should find yourself depressed or contemplating suicide, please get professional help. Please tell someone--a friend, family member, physician, or trusted clergy. Some issues are just too big to take on by yourself. To talk with a trained counselor, call the National Suicide Prevention Lifeline at 1-800-273-8255 (TALK).
I am sharing my tested methods only. My experiences are not to be taken as a substitute for professional help.

I had never been one to feel depressed. I have now felt some serious lows since the EMF wireless radiation poisoning event. I did not know how all-encompassing this depression would be when I first became ill. I had not connected my depression to EHS, until I read online that it is a symptom. Depression is just as much a symptom as is anxiety, confusion, and feelings of fight or flight. Knowing it was a symptom of EHS made it feel more acceptable to me. It didn't make me any happier, but it made it more tolerable.

In my EHS, I am faced with not being able to do the things I used to do. Just to travel like a normal person would be wonderful, instead of always lugging around, or wearing a metalized outfit. I am facing the world in a metalized veil, which is not my first choice, and this in itself is stressful. It makes me depressed to not be able to shop, or be independent. I miss my friends and family, and the ability to meet them in a public venue is now out of bounds due to EMF. I miss my old life. Then there is the ever-present "Why me? Why this? Why now?" The questions that EHS offer are not answerable. The health issues are not one that can be repaired with a shot, pills, therapy, or surgery. In fact, I am a healthy person. Others make me ill with their wireless devices. There is guilt in the financial burden we now face to shield a whole house from EMF. And what if I had to work? These are huge issues that would make anyone depressed. As I did not feel compelled to get professional help or therapy, I decided to explore what I could accomplish on my own against depression. This is what I learned.

First, I learned from my mother. From very young, whenever I told my mom I was feeling sad, she would tell me that I did not have enough to do. I would promptly be given a household chore. As a result, I learned never to tell anyone I was sad unless I wanted to clean house. To this day I am a bad housekeeper. "If you are sad, get busy and stop feeling sorry for yourself" was my lesson early in life. Would a therapist tell me this? I doubt it, but it seemed to work at the time.

In my investigations, I learned that depression can be triggered by genetic predisposition, environmental, or seasonal factors such as SAD (Seasonal Affective Disorder), and chemical imbalance among others. There was not a lot I could find to help with my depression, as I refuse to take prescription drugs or see a therapist. I felt that I did not need another problem or financial cost. What I found out, quite by accident, was certain foods triggered or made my depression worse. I noticed that about an hour after I ate my favorite fix of dark chocolate, I became depressed. I also felt "I want something and I don't know what it is." Well, I wasn't about to do without chocolate, so I experimented with different chocolate bars until I found an organic bar, without the sugars and refinements. (what a fun experiment!) My bouts of depression did not go away but at least I'm not bringing them upon myself as often. So, my lesson learned is that sometimes we have control over a symptom. After my chocolate experiment, I did a search on "foods that trigger depression" and learned that many foods might bring on depression. Depression can be triggered by nutritional deficiencies, and I have read that Vitamin B supplements help. I also take Vitamin D. Many of the foods noted to bring on depression (processed meats, high fructose, corn syrup, dairy products, and coffee) are not ones I eat anyway. I have to be careful in not trying to soothe myself with food.

Sometimes I can feel overwhelmed, a victim, and this sadness leads in turn to my cessation of communicating with others, as I don't want to share the pain. When you have EHS or a multiple chemical sensitivity, there are not many who understand what you are going through. Many don't have someone to talk out situations or problems, but I am lucky in that I have my husband, Eric. If you are a shepherd of a survivor of EHS, please practice at being a good listener.

Right now, writing about this whole EMF poisoning curse is helping me get it outside myself. I can hold it away from me. For some reason, it looks smaller. Art helps, also. I have experimented with ceramics, mosaics, acrylics, and watercolors. I went online and pulled up wet-wooling class, and made two winter wool hats. My favorite art is collage; cutting pictures out that evoke a feeling and gluing them together on a larger piece of board. I enjoy the search for an image that matches a feeling and glomming it with other feelings. I can keep the art or destroy it as if purging. Most art classes are now off limits to me, as they have WiFi and the local art center is unable (or unwilling) to turn it off.

There is much written about music therapy for depresssion. I am at a state that when I hear music, I tend to cry, as it reminds me of what I can no longer do. Of course, this is rock music and it reminds me of rock concerts I used to be able to attend. I should probably be listening to Baroque music, as I have read that it creates an alpha mental state due to its 60 beats a minute. "When your brain wave activity slows down to between 7 and 14 HZ, you are said to be in an alpha state. It is considered a "relaxed" state of mind that allows you to be more receptive, open, creative, and less critical. Edison, Einstein, and many other brilliant thinkers considered a daily ritual of accessing an alpha state of mind essential to their work."
https://www.mindtosucceed.com/alpha-state-of-mind.html

Another thing that helps my depression is grounding, and my favorite way of accomplishing this is to work in the garden. I like to get dirt under my fingernails, pull weeds, turn over the soil, sit cross-legged on the ground. Eric and I, also volunteer at the local botanical gardens. There are no EMFs there, and the work and wildlife, camaraderie and plants all help with my attitude and outlook. Working in the garden can be very creative, and I believe it to be cathartic. Walking on a beach, if one is available, is grounding, and salt water is a good detox.

It helps my mindset if I feel I'm a contributing member of society. This is extremely difficult if I can't be out *in* society. I have found a local non-profit that I love; they have been very successful in stopping logging in the local flood plain. I have been a volunteer secretary for the past several years and feel a part of that success. Sadly, I haven't been able to attend any meetings, as they are held in a room with a wireless router. There are other places I can remotely volunteer, such as the dowsing association or the botanical garden, where I can help with mailings. I suggest finding a group and calling and see if there is any way you can be a participant from home. Many groups would love another set of hands/eyes and spirit to aid in their efforts. It doesn't hurt to ask.

I feel less depressed and better mentally when*:*
- My body feels healthy, I feel better physically. I try to make sure I eat good, organic mostly, food, plenty of water, and supplements
- I have had good night's sleep. Sometimes it takes Melatonin.
- I exercise, either to DVD or by taking walks in nature. I find that gyms have WiFi. I have to force myself to exercise, but always feel better afterwards.
- I am Grounded. I walk at the beach barefoot, close to or in the water, or in my garden.

- I have something to look forward to, plan a vacation/trip. Where is your dream vacation? Plot it on a map, look it up in a book or online.
- I sit in the sun. Natural vitamin D is supposed to help with mood. If there has been a lack of sun, I take supplements.
- I am being creative. To help myself, I set the project up on a table, all ready for my mood to change to a more creative one.
- Journal your journey. In words or through art, it enables me to get it outside of myself and stand farther back.
- It helps to have a sense of accomplishment, so I find it important to make a to-do list. We do so many little things all day, and we are busy, but as the achievements seem small, I hadn't been writing them down. Now, I write them all down. I have felt so depressed that a shower was an accomplishment, so put them all on the list: shower, make bed, and put on earrings. This does two things: it gets it outside of myself so I don't have to lay awake and think about it, and it also puts it in an order. I may not do anything on the list, but I know what I need to accomplish to feel better about the circumstance.

  Make a list of "Things I need to do to protect myself." Make a list of the "Issues I want to learn" and while learning them, take notes. Make another list of "People I need to tell, or ask for help in accomplishing my new list of tasks." (Do not only put one person on this list.) I consider my list making as "getting my ducks in a row." With EHS and the myriad of ways to help yourself, these lists will add structure and control and help you accomplish a semblance of order to your new way of life. Another site that has helped me tremendously is www.emfsafetynetwork.org.
- What matters to you?

Volunteer / Find a need / Find a fight / Take a stand
Read to the young, visit an elder.
- A change of scenery helps lift my mood. Even a short drive in the car to take a walk or get the mail. A ride behind Eric on the motorcycle, feeling the thrill of adrenaline on curvy roads, always helps, no matter how deep the depression.
- Plant something / call someone / write a letter.
- Escapism always works for me. I thank my Mom for instilling in me a love of books. Getting lost in books has given me a great form of escapism that can be embraced late at night or in travel or lying in my Faraday cage. Reading can take me back in time, to new worlds, instill new creative ideas that I most likely won't act on, and even gift refreshing thoughts and inspiration. Keep a good book handy.
- Amazon has been a great help. Everyone has heard of retail therapy. Well, I can't go into stores, but Amazon can grant any wish I have within two days, be it a gift for myself, for someone else, or just tea and biscuits. I should have bought stock in Amazon years ago.
- Positive Affirmations. When I had breast cancer, I had the good fortune to be in the care of a wonderful physician's assistant. He taught me an affirmation technique that I believe greatly expanded my chances of living through breast cancer. I also use this technique when I am depressed. If a mirror is available, look yourself in the eyes and talk to your soul. (If a mirror is not available, ground yourself and look inward). Tell yourself:
You are wonderful. You are strong. You are resilient. You are happy. You are compassionate. (fill in other affirmations that you feel strongly about.) I Love You.

Positive Affirmations are important for everyone to hear.

I read where all the members of a church group-- I believe there were about 20-- wrote their problems on a piece of paper. They put this paper on a table in the middle and then were given a chance to choose a different problem. None chose a different problem, as they were familiar and knew better how to deal with their own problems than others. I don't think I'd keep my problem, but I'd be nosey enough to want to know what others were dealing with, and if they'd want to trade places with me.

My husband, Eric, always tries to fix things and make them better for me. EHS is not one that he can fix, but he has done so much to make it more comfortable and easier to deal with, by offering all his support and just by being available for a hug. There are sites online saying how healthy hugs are for everyone (search "are hugs healthy?"). I think that those who give and receive great hugs knew this before anyone told them. Sometimes, though, when I am feeling especially depressed, I also feel prickly and don't want to be hugged. Eric understands this too, and offers to get me out of the house; a new view or a drive helps also.

Without Eric's help, without his force-feeding me, shopping for groceries or making me take walks, I'd be in worse shape in all respects. I am now totally dependent on Eric to do all chores that are in an area of EMF. I admire the bravery of those with EHS that face this monster alone. Facing all the things I can't do is often overwhelming. Being poisoned by wireless radiation is life altering. Like any harrowing experience, surviving this EMF poisoning has totally changed my perspectives. I believe that most survivors have had to learn to deal with it alone, at least at first. When there is no one to share what is happening, relate to, or be supportive and understanding, you are faced with feeling overwhelmed. Where does one start? You have to gather your personal strength and resilience, and remember that you are not alone. Contact others that have EHS. If you need to ask questions or chat with others: www.es-forum.com .

Those EHS sufferers that have found a way to live independently and with minimal social interaction are true survivors and heroes. I would like to thank all those who helped me when I had so many questions. I would like to thank all those who took the time to answer my calls and emails with support and insight.

Eric's Perspective
by Eric Mills

The first physician I spoke with about my wife's sudden debilitating illness was Dr. Heinlein, the chief physician at the University of Wuerzburg Klinikum in Coburg, Germany. Dr. Heinlein related his son's electromagnetic field exposure to a simple cordless phone and the direct ill effects on his son's wellbeing. Soon after, we were seen by Dr. Horst Eger, a general practitioner in the local village of Naila. He was knowledgeable with wireless exposure and opened our eyes to just how extremely high the radiation readings were that we had been exposed to. It was shocking to hear the much bigger picture portrayed by Dr. Eger. The wireless radiation levels measured at our home greatly exceeded 20,000,000 microwatts per square meter. These outrageous exposure levels had happened week after week, month after month from October 2006 through April 2007, until we moved away from the hilltop house. Through Dr. Eger, we learned of the long-term health concerns, one of the worst being permanent sensitivity to EMF. There are many well-documented studies showing damage to humans at significantly lower levels than what we had been exposed to. Dr. Eger gave Anne a diagnosis of Electromagnetic Hypersensitivity. We had a name to go with the malady.

It became apparent that it was common knowledge within German medical circles of widespread illnesses directly associated with cell towers and wireless devices. The year before we moved to Bavaria, a local German physician, Dr. Cornelia Waldmann-Selsam, had escalated radiation concerns directly to the prime minister of Germany, Dr. Edmund Stoiber. Representing 155 physicians from Oberfranken, she wrote, "a most urgent evaluation of severe health damage caused by pulsed high frequency electromagnetic fields (Mobile telephone base stations, DECT telephones, W-LAN, Bluetooth etc.) far beneath the recommended limit values." Oberfranken is a small region in the northern portion of Bavaria and the very region we had moved to. Local doctors had been trying to escalate attention of the authorities to this major health issue that they were seeing in their patients.

I do not suffer from EHS, though during the poisoning I also experienced health issues, such as nosebleeds, hair falling out, upset stomach, and poor sleep. We had no idea what was happening to us and attributed the ill symptoms to change in climate and diet. I was at work all day while Anne was at home, in close proximity to the cell towers. The exposure did impact me, but nothing approaching Anne's reaction. A couple of medical and scientific experts in the field of EMF radiation have conveyed that Anne is the most sensitive victim that they have ever met. I think this happened because her perceptive nature made her more reactive to these unnatural energies, perhaps due to her prior training as a Reiki Master, a form of hands on healing.

Some progress is being made in Europe to minimize the public's exposure to electromagnetic wireless radiation. France has official White Zones and has removed WiFi from some schools and libraries. New rules have also been enacted restricting children from using cell phones. In comparison, for the most part, the American public is totally unaware of how wireless works and the adverse health effects it causes.

The symptoms of EHS are well documented and I have observed Anne exhibit those very responses when exposed to EMF. Having reviewed the results of hundreds of studies showing health damage and knowing that there are thousands more studies, it is very frustrating to see no coverage of this issue in the public media. None! We might see a television news story report on insomnia and sleeping disorders, but never once does it mention EMF. The American Academy of Pediatrics has seen an explosion of childhood learning disabilities and are pushing the FCC for tighter regulations. We still don't see coverage in the mainstream media covering this issue. Huge increase in heart issues for the young, with no mention of EMF. American doctors with no consideration for the environmental effects on their patients, simply handing out drugs for the various symptoms exhibited. Something has to change. With all the new fears from the rollout of 5G, maybe public recognition of EMF is improving.

I've become jaded by it all. With what I now know, it's all about the money. It's not just a conspiracy. It's a crime. Anne and I have been forced to move time after time, simply to live in a safe place. Over the eight years living in this rural community, the EMF levels have steadily worsened. Two new cell towers are being planned for our little town of less than five hundred. WiFi antennas on the top of nearly every business, just like the neighboring town erected a few years ago. More and more places that had been safe for Anne, are no longer. Less than a quarter mile from our home, a redwood tree now supports many antenna for neighborhood line-of-sight WiFi. Thankfully we have huge trees blocking that signal. More shielding to the house will probably be necessary soon. We live in fear every time we see a telecommunication truck in our neighborhood. At what point do we consider our community no longer safe? And where can we go if we must leave?

I know that Anne hopes that getting this story out there might in some way help others understand the dangers and what steps can be taken to protect themselves. I know we have done more than most in not only protecting ourselves but in trying to help others become aware of EHS. Most folks that suffer from EHS have no choice but to become hermits, hiding in the shadows, isolated from the world of wireless everything. We have continued to travel, camp, hike, enjoy motorcycle trips, but it is getting ever more difficult. Away from EMF Anne is fine and healthy, but radiation levels that she could once tolerate, she can no longer. When Anne does have a minor exposure, it can manifest itself as a sharp headache or sudden onset of aches and pains. If severe enough, numb mindedness can set in for a few hours. In the worse cases, it has quickly led to a loss of vocabulary and motor skills. In nearly all instances, it triggers a "fight or flight" response. I've seen it play out many times and it is scary. I can't help to wonder, just how many of these exposures can she cope with before these symptoms fail to subside.

Since this poisoning, Anne has been unable find a safe place to work. Even being a volunteer is difficult. Her time at the community center is only possible because we unplug the WiFi router and all the other volunteers are nice enough to turn off their phones. I think it is important for me to be a spokesperson for Anne, explaining the medical situation to others that she interacts with. If they show interest, I detail what had happened to her, examples of her symptoms, the findings of scientific studies, or our own personal experiences.

It is important for the caregiver or guardian of an EHS survivor to keep an upbeat attitude. I found it is important for us to focus and celebrate on the little successes and to try not to have obstacles get us down. Occasionally we find a garage sale or an out of the way corner of some event where the EMFs are weak enough for her. We keep trying new venues and somehow find ways to cope when it doesn't work out. All too often we find that the radiation levels are just too high and we've got to get out. I know I need to do a better job of suppressing my own frustrations, work on being more positive, and be less reactive to bad situations. When socializing takes place in safe surroundings, Anne can have the feeling of normalcy without the constant distraction of always having to be aware of EMF. I believe that working to improve that mindset and keeping a healthy perspective is extremely important.

All too often we hear of partners of EHS suffers that are not willing to limit their use of wireless devices. Many simply don't believe that the health concerns are valid. We have found that most EHS sufferers are women, and I think it's important that they have strong support at home. I see shielding Anne as my job. First and foremost, make your home a safe haven from EMF. I've also learned that you can't stay at home all the time. The challenges in travel have made coping with the limitations on our freedom difficult. It is vital to find a means for safe travel and I have written a chapter regarding how to shield your vehicle. Learning how to be an EMF bodyguard for your EHS partner is a required role. I find myself so acquainted with the radiation meter that I can almost perceive the radiation fields in my mind's eye. I am always looking for elevated radiation levels and where the exposure levels might be less. I am always totally focused on our surroundings, being constantly aware of who just entered the room and if the meter shows increased radiation. The lack of support networks for those EHS survivors and families is a concern. As a husband of an EHS survivor and a disabled wife, I don't really have anyone to reach out to, or speak to about this. There is no support circle for caregivers that I'm aware of.

I really don't like the word caregiver, and I don't see myself in that role, nor do I see Anne as an invalid. Sure, there are the everyday errands that she used to enjoy, but can no longer do, like shopping and going to the post office. Maybe I'm more of a shepherd, being there for her in other ways, like when she experiences fight or flight, and becomes confused about what has happened. Sometimes it is explaining to others their need to turn off their phones so that she doesn't have to leave. Occasionally its little things, like getting her out of the house before she goes nuts or simply encouraging her to get back to her artwork or gardening.

There are tough challenges, too, like finding or forcing access to a medical environment that is safe for her. Our recent success in working through the county's ADA Compliance Office has allowed Anne to now safely utilize the county book mobile. This was a big win for us and something I hope we can build on. By demanding ADA accommodations, maybe we can improve access to medical services and public entertainment in our community. Perhaps I should be more willing to join community organizations and be a voice in driving change.

I also need to look to the future for what challenges we might be faced with. What happens if I were to have a medical emergency? I know Anne would want to be with me, but we can't have such an event become a major exposure for her. At least I have confidence in the full-body personal shielding outfit that has shown to be effective. Something that I would like Anne to do is to accept wearing her protective clothing out in public. She is less self-conscious wearing it while shopping, but only if we are out of town where no one recognizes her.

The current situation with ever-expanding sources of EMF is unacceptable; so are the falsehoods of the wireless industry concerning safety, the ignorance of politicians, and the willingness of the public to accept anything wireless. "Big Wireless" has been very successful at suppressing what is truly happening. That is the struggle, to turn the tide of regulations influenced by entrenched industry forces resisting any notion of adverse health effects of non-ionizing radiation. We can hopefully have some influence; but we can't possibly change it with all the big money behind it. This is society's fight and I don't see society having any willingness to change.

I am really looking forward to the book being finished, as Anne has to keep reliving the pain and sadness. Once done, she can get back to her gardening. I know she is happiest getting dirt under her fingernails and grounding herself barefoot in backyard.

Eric Mills

Intervention for EHS Access

Living with Electromagnetic Sensitivities, like any environmental illness, is difficult with all the modern-day conveniences and chemicals. Following are several examples of how Eric and I were able to work around obstacles to accomplish our goals.

When Eric and I found out that I would be needing surgery for breast cancer and stomach issues, we were faced with the possibility that I would have difficulty finding a safe place to recuperate while in the hospital. Our meters have shown us that hospitals have pervasive EMF Radiation. Eric approached the hospitals facility manager and told them of my issue with EMFs and how it was imperative that I be in a room free of radiation. The hospital did an amazing job of providing us with a room where they removed all wireless devices. They also made sure this room was away from the nurses' break room, which held the microwave oven. The nurses put signs on the door for all those entering to turn off their cell phones or leave them outside the room. For a different procedure, in a different hospital, when they could not get a room without other patients and their cell phones, they made an ICU room available for our use.

***

Visiting a doctor's office can be painful. My visits to my oncologist always led to many EHS symptoms such as hot flashes, nausea, tunnel vision, and 'fight or flight'. At times, I knew the doctor was asking a question, but I had no idea what he was saying, and I couldn't form thoughts into words for a response. At this point, I experienced fight or flight, a noted symptom of EHS, and ran out of the room. In leaving, I realized I didn't know where to go and didn't know where I was. I just had to get away. Eric found me and guided me to our vehicle and we drove home. Eric contacted the Sutter Health building manager, and together they surveyed the entire three-story building with our radiation meter. It took them a couple hours, but they found an area designated for conferences on the third floor that had low EMF. My doctor now holds our visits in this EMF free White Zone, a huge conference room, where they have placed one chair and one gurney bed.

***

I needed an ophthalmologist, as my glasses needed replacing, but our rural area does not have one. Eric started searching, riding his motorcycle to ophthalmology offices throughout the county. He would test the ambient radiation in their office with our meter to see if I could be a patient. All of the ophthalmologist offices had readings that would have made me ill. One office I called stated they did not have Wifi. I made an appointment, we drove the hour and a half to get there. We discovered that their office was half a block from a giant cell phone tower and the radiation almost pegged the meter. We finally found an ophthalmologist about a year later. Here there were no cell towers and the radiation was not quite so high, but high enough that it still mandated I wear my full head protective metalized clothing. (>1.25 V/m). It was a surprise when the doctor told us that I was not his only patient with EHS, and he was familiar with the illness and its symptoms.

***

Being so rural, we have a two-hour drive to a hospital. This means that if I had an emergency, I would have to use our little local health clinic. I know from previous visits that the EMF have gotten steadily worse as they add more wireless devices to their patient rooms. The radiation in our local clinic is now extreme (>3.45 V/m). In the waiting room, they encourage cell phones with a sign advertising free WiFi. Upon entering, every patient has their face in their smart phone. Rain or shine, I must wait outside until my appointment. I called the building manager and told her my experiences and asked if there was any way they could put aside an area that was away from any wireless or had a much less negative impact on my person. As I already explained, this is called a White Zone where there are no

EMFs for those who are sensitive, and I believe that all medical facilities should have one available. I told her I would appreciate being able to have a doctor visit or see the emergency medics without having so much physical response to their wireless devices. As no one had ever suggested that to her, she asked a few questions and said she would have to contact her superiors. Eric wrote her a letter and attached a link where she could get more information about how other hospitals had mitigated the issue. We received an email letter response from her superior, bringing up the issue of a room that is rented for meetings. I have no idea what this had to do with me seeing a physician in their facility. The answer I was given had nothing to do with the issues I brought forth in my asking for a safe place to see my physician pain free. How are we going to handle this? How can a doctor take a true blood pressure when the rooms EMF negatively impact that reading? My heart beat elevates when confronted by a certain frequency, but that is not my normal heart beat. I am going to ask for a physician house call.

***

We get calls from local people that are ill asking Eric if he would check the EMF radiation in their home or work environment. Ever willing to help, Eric goes to their home with the radiation meters and spends time, free of charge, going through their living space. He finds offensive radiation and explains how they could go about mitigating the problem. Wired phones, wired computers, wire mesh over smart meters, etc. Eric always brings a corded phone. In this way, he can show them the sky-high radiation readings before he unplugs their cordless DECT phones and again after he attaches a corded phone. They now have a choice. Eric spends an hour or more at their home or workplace on their request. It is disheartening to later learn they don't follow through with any of his suggestions. At one home, Eric suggested the couple install wire mesh around their smart meter and move wireless equipment out of their bedrooms. They did this, but instead of giving symptoms a couple days to dissipate, when an immediate health change did not happen overnight, they moved the equipment back in. In one home check, Eric suggested the person replace his cordless phone with a corded phone, which he did, but then purchased blue tooth for his vehicle! People seem to want their conveniences over their health.

***

We have learned that the front section of stores are always high in EMF radiation. The registers, the ATM machines, the lottery machines are all emitting radiation. I found that I couldn't enter one of the local grocery stores without feeling "thick-lipped," tunnel vision, and confusion. The radiation meter readings were greater than 4.5 V/m, which is quite high. Eric approached the store owner, showing his findings and explaining that it not only kept me from shopping but that this was hazardous to his employees. That went nowhere. I can no long do any grocery shopping. In this rural area, there are not many choices. I am now in a situation that if Eric goes out of the area for any length of time, I can't shop for myself without wearing metalized protective gear.

***

We have the most wonderful dentist in our area. We are especially lucky because he is not only a skilled dentist, but is supportive in my EHS issues. When we go into his office, he asks his assistants to turn off their cell phones. He asks those in the adjoining rooms and in the waiting room to turn their phones off also. He knows that it is to both our benefits for me to feel well during my visit.

***

We pay, through taxes, for the library system, but due to my EHS and the large readings of EMF in the library, we are unable to take advantage of what a library has to offer. Eric wrote a letter to the county library, explaining our situation. Eric explained what EHS was, and what symptoms I experienced when we tried to use the library and bookmobile. Eric asked that there be a way for me to use the library in a safe way. He asked that we be able to go to the bookmobile either as last or first patron, and that all wireless devices be turned off. The county library responded with a "yes," and set up dates and times where I could safely use their book mobile. This is great!

***

I needed to update my driver's license. I called to Department of Motor Vehicles and explained the EHS situation. They offered to let me be the first or the last customer, my choice, with all cell phones turned off. They explained that, due to security issues, all of DMV computers are wired. This was so accommodating and appreciated.

***

I needed to purchase a vehicle and found one I liked online. The car lot happened to be located in a big city. We drove to the lot that was selling the car, but we found the radiation was >4.5 V/m, which is nearly fifty times more than I can comfortably endure. Eric explained the issues and the salesman was nice enough to help us look for a safe space with low radiation levels throughout the compound. We were lucky enough to find a small closet in an unused area of the building with much lower EMF. We brought a chair and lights, and I bought my car in a closet!

***

The town next door has a wonderful little pub that Eric and I frequented weekly for a couple years. The owner, due to customer demand, decided to put in WiFi. I would now no longer be able to belly up to the bar or meet my friends for the evening. Eric and I explained our situation to Tim, the owner. Being such a wonderful person, Tim declared Mondays "No WiFi" day; he gave me a day in his establishment! I could enjoy the ambiance and friendships on Mondays. If someone came in with a cell phone, he would ask them to turn it off. When my birthday came around, Tim put my name on the marquis, stated no wireless or cell phones for the evening, and I invited all my friends and a band. It was a great night and a fun party. We give our heartfelt thanks to Tim, the owner of the little brick pub, for his understanding and support. Due to the addition of numerous WiFi 'hot spots' throughout town, we are no longer able to enjoy this great pub as radiation comes in through the front window.

So I have learned to be proactive where not only my health is concerned but in areas where there is a chance to remain an active and contributing member of society.

The New Normal

How does one explain "new normal"? I am a healthy and regular person that now, due to Electromagnetic Field radiation from wireless devices, I have a new normal way of living. There are conflicting estimates on what percent of the population suffers from EHS and are having to find a new normal. There have been studies suggesting a range between 5 to 35% of the population have the syndrome.

When we first moved to this rural area in 2011, I lived normally. The cell phone reception was virtually non-existent and the local coffee house had a sign reading "No WiFi." The theatre, the shops, and the fishing pier were all free of radiation and open for me to enjoy safely. Now, our small rural town has line of sight WiFi. Many buildings sport cell antenna, so even a walk through town is off limits. All stores now have WiFi Hot Spots and wireless devices. Eric and I used to frequent a local fishing pier, meet friends at the pub, and watch fishing boats come in with their hauls. We used to be monitors along a bluff walk, and volunteers at Cinco de Mayo celebrations and fund raising events. I used to frequent the local art center, take classes, and enjoy their music and art venue. I used to be a participant in the Women's March, worked as a judge at a yearly car show, and participant in The Lions Club. In other words, I was an active and contributing member of the community. If an opportunity presented itself, I would try to partake. Due to the higher EMF I am confronted with at every turn, I am now cloistered at home.

There are many times when I must get out of the house; when I need a change of pace and place. On occasion, my husband has been able to find us a little pub with an outside patio area that has low EMF. In these few instances, we enjoy a beer or glass of wine, but most times it is limited by the arrival of other customers with their cell phones. Lately, I have been reticent to delve into new experiences, as they have ended in disappointment. My hopeful expectations become dashed upon the realization that our promised venue is all EMF*d up. What starts as fun preparations, getting dressed up, and anticipating has ended in a washout. What makes trying to live normally an act of activism, is the hundreds of discussions about EMF radiation we have had with others in the process of us asking them to turn their phones off. We explain the situation with my sensitivity to EMFs and give them one of our information cards. I made business-size information cards that list symptoms and where they can get more information on EMF/EHS. People are usually pretty nice, turning off their phones. Every so often we are blessed with new friends and enjoy new scenery.

Trying to be in public around unknowing (or uncaring) people means we are confronted with their attempt to reason or dampen their own fear. Though there are literally thousands of peer-reviewed scientific studies showing the solid validity of EMF negative impacts on health, there are still those people that do not believe that you have anything other than a creative imagination. Even some physicians, regarding EHS, still say "it is all in your head." EMFs are just one more invisible monster that many feel they have no control over, so they don't even want to think about. For some, a smart phone is their whole life. We have observed teenagers clutch their phones close to their chest when not looking at the screen. We've watched as this all-important phone distracts them driving, from friends, walking in traffic or crowds, to a point of calamity.

In speaking of EHS or wearing my metalized clothing I have been confronted with ridicule, disbelief, and open-mouthed amazement. I believe that in reality many people are in fear of the things they can't see or can't be in control of, so they deny them. How can they fight what they can't see? They don't have to fight if they don't believe. This ignorance of the populace can only come to a stop if those who have EHS start becoming more visible. Those of us with EHS should try to be more vocal. We need to teach those in the community that show interest that there is another dimension that encompasses us all: man-made pulsed microwave radiation, and it adversely affects everyone: us, them, their family, pets, and our natural environment.

I don't look forward to watching life being experienced by others through the window, with no chance of joining. I keep trying different venues because there is always the chance that we meet new and open people. There are those successes that let me pretend, for a minute, that I am normal; that Eric can pretend all is well. I guess that's why I keep trying to be social. Following are some of the positives and a few negatives we experienced in looking for safe venues, dealing with those without EHS, how we have been welcomed or judged, and how we have handled the situations as we try to live normally. I am sure that those with EHS can relate.

***

The next town over has a lovely community center where Eric and I have enjoyed their gatherings and breakfasts. Occasionally, we have volunteered to work their benefits. On one occasion, in offering to work a crab feed, we discovered that WiFi had been installed. We told the management of our situation and how we would like to volunteer with their benefit. The management was nice enough to unplug the router, and in addition, they asked everyone to turn off their cell phones. Eric and I were able to spend a couple of hours being social and lend our help. We were invited back for the breast cancer fund drive. This was so generous of the management and we made sure they knew we appreciated the gesture by supporting them at every chance. It goes to show, that it doesn't hurt to ask others for their understanding and unplug the wireless devices.

***

Eric and I found that a local restaurant had a patio area with a couple of nice Adirondack chairs and no present EMF. We would go about once a week and enjoy a beer in the sun. Invariably, someone would come to sit beside us, and usually they were nice enough to turn their phones off. Of the people we met there, Americans for the most part were not familiar with

EHS or the dangers of EMF. On the other hand, those that were visiting from Europe were not only knowledgeable about EMF, but turned their phones off of their own volition after they heard I had EHS! In one instance the young 10-year-old daughter of a visiting German couple was the one that asked others to turn their phones off.

***

I am a volunteer at a thrift shop, and strive to make sure that I am seen as a hard worker. I want to be considered an asset, as I am asking my co-workers to turn off their cell phones. The women and men I work with are all aware of my problem. They seem to like me and don't mind turning off their phones in exchange for my help. They are all very nice in this way. There has been occasion when I start to feel ill; nausea, hot flashes, tunnel vision, numbness, confusion, faltering balance, and spiky headaches. In my effort to leave, my co-workers realize the problem and are so kind as to make sure all present check their phones to make sure they are off. Once I feel ill enough to have to leave, fight or flight takes over. I am in no physical or mental state to be able to argue, explain, or stand up for myself. Usually when I get to a point of having to leave, I have left it too long, and am ill for the remainder of the day with vertigo, flu symptoms, and general malaise. I often feel very depressed after such experiences, and I don't know if it is a symptom, or I am just sad that I had to leave something I enjoyed. I consider myself blessed to have such wonderful co-workers.

***

Eric and I had joined a group of volunteers to walk a well-used hiking trail several times a week to pick up trash left by tourists. We enjoyed doing this for a several years. This was a way I could help the community and it was in an area of our locale that was safe from EMF radiation. Sadly, when WiFi antennas were erected on the tops of local businesses throughout town, we had to discontinue.

***

I was a board member for the local community center and a secretary during their meetings. This was a position I really enjoyed. The other members were aware of my EHS health issues, and were very nice about turning off their cell phones. Due to requests from several members, the board members decided to put in WiFi throughout the community center property. As a courtesy to me, they had the console constructed in a way that enabled us to have the ability to turn off the WiFi if I was in the vicinity. So nice! I always bring my meter with me, and one day found that the radiation readings in our meeting office had become too high for me to be comfortable. I discovered that this was due to the hotel across from the center installing a new antenna that now emitted radiation into our meeting room. I could no longer hold the board member and secretarial position.

***

Eric and I love to hike, and have joined in hikes over the years with a local club. We have had problems with members leaving their phones on during the hike, but wanted the social aspects so thought we'd try another hike. We decided to participate in a hike in the nature preserve with the club. Sadly, there were people on this hike that had cell phones with large radiation output (4.5 V/m) that even though they were not expecting a call, refused to turn their phone off. We had to be apart from the social aspect of the group and walk by ourselves. There was no radiation on the one and a half mile uphill climb, until we got closer to the top and I started feeling ill. We found that right where we were supposed to eat, hanging over the picnic tables, stood a large cell antenna with radiation readings from a quarter mile away of over 1.5 V/m. As this was a new park, the antenna had not yet made the www.antennasearch.com listing. We walked down the steep hill quickly. I sent a letter to the facilitator of the hiking club explaining EHS and symptoms. The facilitator was wonderful in her understanding, and the next hike she organized, she actually announced in the invite that this would be a "no cell phone" hike, as someone in the group had a sensitivity. All attendees were to leave their cell phone in their autos. Her kind action is appreciated.

***

Two years ago, I entered a new local store, but found I was unable to shop due to extreme high (>3.0 V/m) EMF readings on my meter. I showed the owner the readings and the fact that he could get rid of the radiation just by changing out his DECT phone to a corded phone. He refused and was not interested in any information as he did not believe in radiation being harmful. I did not push the issue, but wished I could have shopped at his establishment. Recently, this same man contacted me, requesting help in fighting a new cell tower that will be erected a mile from his new home. I am pretty sure that this cell tower would surround him with less wireless radiation than his cordless phone emits, and he sits next to his phone every day.

***

I am a dowser. Though dowsers search for many things, I mainly dowse for water. I became a dowser at the suggestion of one of my doctors. To this end, I took many classes and lessons from local dowsing mentors. This is my attempt to turn lemons into lemonade. With my sensitivities I can help others. Usually my jobs are in very rural areas, but this particular request was for a job in town. In order to build they needed water. I found myself in a situation where I could not get a good reading with my dowsing sticks; two copper L-shaped rods. This had never happened before. I believe the dowse was being influenced by the radiation soup I found myself from cell antenna on nearby roofs. The rods would swing in wild arches, as if overwhelmed. The rods also seemed to follow vehicles on the nearby road. I believe the rods were following the vehicles' radiation. In the years dowsing, I had never had that happen and never since. I do not believe I can dowse in a town. Give me rural any day.

***

Refreshingly, those we have met lately have been forthcoming with experiences of their own regarding EHS, and have intelligent questions regarding EMF. Occasionally, we do meet those who still have misconceptions of a cell phone. For instance, many don't know that when the reception is bad, their phone ramps up the radiation in order to be able to connect with the cell tower. If in an area of poor reception or in their vehicle, your phone is EMF*ing up the whole area in its attempt to keep in constant tag with the tower. Their cell phone is sending out constant spikes of EMFs. We have also found that some people don't know how to turn their phones off. They mistakenly believe that turning off the screen turns the phone off. Of note, we have found that in the act of turning off a phone, the phone puts out a huge spike of EMFs causing a huge ramp up of EMF. I must quickly move away whenever someone turns off their cell phone.

***

We had metal signs made that have "Radiation Free Zone" and a "no cell phone" insignia. They read "Please leave cell phones and all wireless devices in your vehicles." We have one sign attached to the front of our home and we keep one sign in our vehicle, used mostly when camping. The "Radiation Free Zone" sign on our home has brought interest from our Fed Ex and UPS drivers. These delivery drivers are marvelous in that I see them actually leaving their wireless communication devices in their vehicles while they walk their delivery to our home. They are nice enough to accept the "Radiation Free Zone" sign literally. I asked them about this, and they told me that we were not the only sensitives on their delivery routes and they extend this gesture to the others as well!

Anne Mills

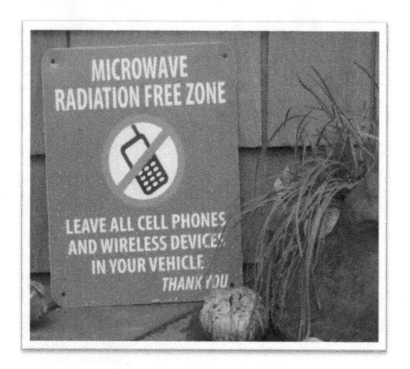

Thank you UPS and FedEx drivers!

***

We were blessed with dear friends visiting. In checking our radiation meter the warning lights started flashing even though our visitors had left their cell phones in their vehicle. These short EMF bursts were read (>3.0 V/m) high on the meter. As we had no idea what was emitting radiation, our friend dumped out her purse, and there, the culprit revealed itself: a small square "Tile" tracking device for keys and luggage.

***

Eric and I are avid sport motorcyclists; well, Eric is the motorcyclist, and I am a skilled and active passenger. This is not a cruiser ride; this is sport riding; the bend over at the corners at speed riding. The rides are thrilling and a total adrenalin rush. We have over forty-years of experience, and have enjoyed many great adventures, both here in the United States and throughout Europe. It has become increasingly difficult for me to ride with Eric, due to the levels of radiation we find everywhere. Eric tries to travel only on rural roads so we don't have to take freeways with their cell tower mast repeaters, but that is not always possible. When we need gas, due to EMFs in towns, Eric has to find a safe place for me and drop me off, returning for me after refueling. It is difficult for me to find a restroom without being bombarded into illness. It is impossible to find someplace to eat without radiation. It has become increasingly difficult to find areas to ride where we are not suddenly faced with a looming cell tower. Our friends with whom we enjoy motorcycling don't mind going out of their way so I can be well on the ride. I am blessed in this way.

***

I was unable to attend my father's funeral and memorial in 2018. The radiation, even with my headgear, was making me ill. I did not have full body clothing protection at the time. If you do not have protective gear, do not put it off. You never know when you will need it. (see chapter on Personal Protection and Protective Clothing.)

***

To safeguard health, I believe that those of us with EHS have an obligation to try and educate those whose company we want to keep, both family and friends. I now view these attempts to have a relationship with family, locals, and society as my form of activism. I think to myself, "well, if this poisoning event happened for a reason, maybe that reason was to raise awareness in those we love." It is my hope that maybe I can protect them from my fate. Your family, close friends, maybe a co-worker were the first souls you told. You shared your symptoms, the harms, and how they can protect themselves. They see the symptoms first hand, they know you; this should make a difference. And for the most part they nod, smile, agree, but many times change nothing! They don't think it applies to them. They think that since only you feel it, it only affects you, and continue to keep one phone in their front pocket and one in their back pocket. If you are an EHS sufferer, and have attempted to help inform those you love, just know you have done what you could; they are addicted, which is a whole other ball game.

***

Luckily, there are those kind and compassionate people, like our neighbors, who believed our story. They believe our stories, lend support, and even burden themselves financially by turning away smart meters so I don't have to sleep in a cage. Good people. There are co-workers who leave their phones in their vehicles. There are people that approach us and tell us that they have cleaned up their homes and feel better and are off their thyroid meds! So for those readers who believe they now suffer from EHS radiation poisoning, I am sorry. Through the encounters we've had, it is always heartening to know that there are many good people that have an open mind and are willing to accept us in our disability. There is no cure or no way to undo the poisoning. In my ventures, I must find ways to help those that need it, and turn lemons into lemonade. Try to get in touch with other EHS survivors through support groups or start your own support group. Know that you are stronger than you think, and know that you are not alone.

Killing us Softly –

5G, Cell towers, Smart meters, WiFi in schools

Frog soup: There is a proverb about boiling a frog. If you put a frog in boiling water, he will jump out. If you put a frog in tepid water and slowly bring it to boil, the frog won't react even when the water starts to boil. The frog has become comfortable in the pot, and will be cooked to death before it realizes what is happening and react to save itself. With the ever increasing amount of radiation being emitted into our environment, are we to suffer the same fate as the frog?

Many believe that EMF radiation is only a problem for those with EHS, without understanding that EMF's affects everyone and every living thing on earth. If microwave radiation can go through a brick wall, it can go through your skin and affect every cell in your body. As we are now becoming enlightened, I feel it is only right that we share that knowledge and help others understand EMF and its dangers.

Writing as a Form of Activism
As travel makes me ill, and being in public places subjects me to Electromagnetic Field wireless radiation, it is extremely difficult to be an activist. This means that my activism must be either in small social gatherings or take the form of writing.

Anne Mills

Schools: Computers, Yes; Wifi, No !

I can't think of anything worse than sending one's children off to school, thinking they are safe, only to have them bombarded by EMF's in their classrooms. What are we thinking? Children are more susceptible to EMF than adults due to their thinner skulls. EMF's have been linked with not only autism and childhood learning disabilities, but many illnesses. You can learn more by going to: www.EHTrust.org or www.wiredchild.org . Our children are the love of our lives and the future of the world. Many teachers are becoming ill from electromagnetic radiation from WiFi and students' cell phones in the classroom. WiFi-supported computers are now mandated in some schools. Get the computers wired. Eric and I went to a bake sale in the local school auditorium and the EMF levels almost peaked the meter! I believe in computers, and enjoy using mine. Every child needs to have computer skills and computers certainly give learning a wonderful dimension, but please wire the computers. Schools have been donated equipment for children from the computer industry that can only be used wirelessly. Are parents OK with this, or just unaware? Many don't realize that upper echelon high tech sector (Gates, Jobs, Zuckerberg) sent their children to low tech schools and limit wireless exposure.
www.chicagotribune.com/lifestyles/ct-learning-without-tech-steve-jobs-balancing-20140918-column.html

Along with radiation in the classrooms from wireless devices, many schools have allowed cell towers to be erected in their playgrounds and on rooftops. The International Association of Firefighters was so concerned about radiation emissions from cell towers atop firehouses, that they commissioned a study that confirmed adverse effects on the firefighters. They then authored a policy statement asking for exemptions from placement of cell towers on their facilities so they could maintain "optimal cognitive and physical capacity at all times." Fire houses are now exempt from sporting a cell tower due to acknowledged ill

health effects, but cell towers are ubiquitous in school playgrounds. How crazy is that? It is All EMF*d Up! There are quite a few schools in Europe and the U.S that have become more cognizant of the negative health effects of their wireless devices in the classrooms and are removing WiFi and cell phone antenna to reduce exposure for their teachers and students. To find out how the schools are accomplishing this feat, go to:
www.ehtrust.org/policy
http://www.parentsforsafetechnology.org/
http://www.wiredchild.org/

The American Academy of Pediatrics, representing 60,000 primary care pediatricians, submitted a letter on August 29, 2013 to the Federal Communications Commission (FCC). The letter "urges the FCC to adopt radiation standards" that 1) protect children's health and well-being from radiation emitted by cell phones and other wireless devices; 2) reflect how people actually use their cell phones; and 3) provide sufficient information that enables consumers to make informed decisions when they purchase mobile phones. The letter is also available on the FCC's web site at
https://ecfsapi.fcc.gov/file/7520941318.pdf

Cell Towers

The Telecommunications Act of 1996 makes it so that citizens can't fight a cell tower installation due to adverse health issues. So that you also don't fight it for aesthetics, cell towers come disguised in a myriad of different species of trees. Cell towers are designed to blend in with their surroundings disguised as everything from a vineyard fan, a cactus, palm tree, a flagpole, or concealed as part of water tanks and billboards. The telecom industry wants you to ignore or be oblivious to what is making you ill. Mounted on these cell towers are cell antenna from a myriad of different companies all transmitting at different frequencies. Small cell antenna can also be attached to any roof or pole or tree, (which eventually kills the tree). Cell towers line all freeways and country roads alike. Cell towers stand proud on hilltops or are hidden in bell towers of a church. The Catholic Church augments donations with money from industry by putting cell phone antenna in their beautiful spires and in their school's grounds. Don't be blind to cell towers and antenna by looking through them. Be aware.

www.electricsense.com/7115/cell-tower-installation-prevention-emfs/

www.parentsforsafetechnology.org

https://www.saferemr.com/2015/04/cell-tower-health-effects.html

If not for a cell tower, I would not have EHS. Cell towers are responsible for countless and irreparable health issues (and I believe deaths) yet to be recognized by mainstream medical. Though we rely on cell towers to make our cell phone/communications work, cell towers are not monitored for radiation emission compliance by independent governance.

Cell towers have been linked to suicide clusters. "THE spate of deaths among young people in Britain's suicide capital could be linked to radio waves from dozens of mobile phone transmitter masts near the victims' homes. Dr Roger Coghill, who sits on a Government advisory committee on mobile radiation, has discovered that all 22 youngsters who have killed themselves in Bridgend, South Wales, over the past 18 months lived far closer than average to a mast [cell tower]. He has examined worldwide studies linking proximity of masts to depression. Dr Coghill's work is likely to trigger alarm and lead to closer scrutiny of the safety of masts, which are frequently sited on public buildings such as schools and hospitals." www.eon3emfblog.net/smeter-moratorium-laws-spread-emfs-suicides-digest-for-3-4-11

Cell towers bring down property value. The National Institute for Science, Law and Public Policy's survey "Neighborhood Cell Towers & Antennas—Do They Impact a Property's Desirability?" initiated June 2, 2014, has now been completed by 1,000 respondents. "The overwhelming majority of respondents (94%) reported that cell towers and antennas in a neighborhood or on a building would impact interest in a property and the price they would be willing to pay for it. And 79% said under no circumstances would they ever purchase or rent a property within a few blocks of a cell tower or antenna." www.takebackyourpower.net and www.emfanalysis.com/property-values-declining-cell-towers .

If you find that you live or work in close proximity to a cell tower, I would suggest 1) getting a meter and determining how much RF you are being exposed to; 2) getting in touch with a building biologist who can make suggestions on how and where you could be using shielding. Eric and I thought we would be safe from EMF in our basement cellar, but found that the radiation from the nearby cell tower came into our basement through a two foot by ten inch window that was at ground level. The radiation had bounced off of the side of the neighbor's house and through the window. Finding how the radiation enters your home or employment is important in how you can protect yourself from it.

"Smart" Utility Meters

The utility companies have now mandated that all their customers have a smart meter to measure energy use. A smart meter is like a little radio station that sends out a short intense blast of EMF Radiation six to twelve times a minute; that is 17,000 times a day. This enables the utility company to bill you more for your use of energy during peak hours. I have not heard of anyone to date that has said that they just love their smart

meter, or that it has saved them money or time. I do not believe that this is the reason a smart meter was designed. I believe that smart meters have been rolled out so that the utility company can have control of your appliances and so they can harvest the date/time info of your usage, data mining for their own use or to sell. They were designed as a means of surveillance. It has become known that smart meters have surge protection only towards the pole and not going towards a home. This has been suggested as the real reason behind many fires. We have seen instances where homes without smart meters are the ones that are left undamaged in the midst of destroyed homes that had smart meters.
https://takebackyourpower.net/1000s-of-smart-meter-fires-new-whistleblower-court-evidence-video/
http://emfsafetynetwork.org/smart-meters/smart-meter-fires-and-explosions/
http://americanfreepress.net/why-are-houses-burning-but-not-trees/
https://www.naturalnews.com/049518_smart_meters_EMF_pollution_utilities.html
http://emfsafetynetwork.org/smud-smart-meter-burn-out-causes-electrical-failure-fire-hazard/

  If you are lucky enough to still have an old analog utility meter with the rotating disk, there are ring locks you can purchase to protect it. In this way, the utility company needs to contact you to remove the ring, and you then have a chance to tell them if you do or do not want a meter. If you find that you do have a smart meter and do not want one, contact your utility company and demand an opt-out of the smart meter. For help fighting a smart utility meter, visit www.emfsafetynetwork.org. I would not accept a non-transmitting or low-transmitting utility unit that the industry has been pushing instead of the old generation analog meter. Though touted as non-transmitting, they have been shown to still transmit EMF. (For personal/home protection against radiation from EMF emitting utility meters, see the chapter on Protecting your Home and Work Environment.)

When the smart meter roll-out began in our region, all our immediate neighbors opted out, just for me and our situation. We are truly blessed to have such wonderful neighbors, as it cost quite a bit of money for the initial opt-out, with a continuing outlay monthly for years after. At our old home in the East Bay, we read our meters for fifteen years, with the utility company coming to our home once a year to verify readings. Once the smart meters were installed, no one in the area was allowed to read their own meter.

Note: Smart gas meters are also being installed, and these also emit radiation.

Our Activism against Smart Meters

The search to live in an area without EMF radiation led to our fifth move in as many years. We found an area that had little or no EMF, but just as we moved in, the smart meters were being rolled out. I believe it is called "rolled out" because they steam roll over any argument you might present and do what they want, even if it is without the owner's permission. Eric and I believe that utility customers have a "right to know," so Eric and I decided to sponsor a meeting so others in our area could learn about all aspects of smart meters, not just what the utility company wanted them to know. Lloyd Morgan is an electrical engineer, an internationally known microwave radiation researcher/educator, and brain tumor survivor. He was nice enough to be our speaker at the meeting. We wrote a letter to the editor of our local paper to try and educate those who were not at the meeting. We believe that it is better that people make informed decisions.

It was only a week or so after our smart meter meeting that I was driving in the neighborhood and noticed a Wellington truck, a contractor for the local power company. The contractor was pulling up to people's homes, entering their closed gates, and replacing their electrical meters without notifying the homeowner. This made me so mad. The next house the driver pulled his truck into, I pulled my car into the gated driveway after him, opened both my car doors, affectively boxing in his vehicle. I went to the driver and asked him if he had knocked on the door and alerted the owner to what he was doing, and he said "no." I told him he needed to do that. He went to the door; the owner opened and told him she did not want a smart meter and she had alerted the utility company to that fact. I suggested the owner contact the sheriff and call the local newspaper. The newspaper representative, Dave, arrived much quicker than the sheriff, and gathered information and took photos. The Wellington smart meter employee wanted to leave, so I left and he did also. The subsequent newspaper article effectively let locals know that smart meters were going in, and unless they let PGE know, unless they took action, they would have a smart meter. www.stopsmartmeter.org

Commercial Awareness

In your new awareness of how pervasive EMF's have become and the growing number of people that are becoming sensitive, you might also start to notice symptoms of acquaintances that sound startlingly familiar. For me, it is so difficult *not* to ask if they have a cordless phone on the head of their bed or live by a cell tower. Now when I watch TV, I am aware of how many pharmaceutical advertisements are for symptoms brought on by EMF's. These drugs target skin issues, eye issues, thyroid issues, heart palpitations, insomnia, depression, and many other EHS symptoms. Who is looking at the cause of these symptoms? Not many are connecting the dots. I notice in commercials the auto companies are touting their vehicles ability to sense other vehicles, actually showing how EMF's surround their vehicle. I notice in commercials how the telecom industry tries to normalize the idea of every child having a cell phone or laptop or how they depict the strength of their wireless device using colors going through walls. Companies are using commercials to normalize robots in our everyday lives by showing robots in living rooms and interacting with families. It is a silent "it's going to happen, get used to it," A.I. of things to come. Once you are aware, you will see the pervasiveness of all things big telecom. It took twenty years for government to protect us against DDT, asbestos, and cigarettes among other things. We don't have twenty years with the now-pervasive EMF. Share your awareness. Vote wisely.

Against 5G

Like the smart meter, 5G small cell antenna are mandated by the FCC and rolled out throughout the country. This is an ultimate act of war against humanity. 5G is a radiation emitting device that has had no research for health and safety ramifications; there are no regulations and there are no safety guidelines. Our governmental agencies of FDA, EPA, and the FCC are not doing anything to protect the U.S. citizens. They know the dangers, as the same frequency is used in Direct Energy Weaponry. The FCC, the body of government that is supposed to be protecting us, is acting on behalf of the wireless industry in speeding up the process of installing 5G by waiving all arguments against. "We, the people" are actually going to be "We, the guinea pigs" for the benefit of industry. The only good thing about 5G is that it has made more people aware of EMF radiation. Everyone should realize that the radiation emitted by 5G is the same as 4G, 3G, and the cell phone they hold to their head. 5G, with it's much higher frequencies, will have significantly higher signal concentration than the current 4G and will require many more antenna to be installed to insure coverage. Antenna will have to be placed on nearly every power pole next to or across the street from every home and business.

The biggest concern is how these new 5G wavelengths will affect the skin, our body's largest organ. "The human body has between two million to four million sweat ducts." Dr. Ben-Ishai of Hebrew University, Israel explains that our sweat ducts act like "an array of helical antennas when exposed to these wavelengths" meaning that we become more conductive. A recent New York study that experimented with 60GHz waves stated that "the analyses of penetration depth show that more than 90% of the transmitted power is absorbed in the epidermis and dermis layer." www.electricsense.com

5G will have extremely high EMF pulsed radiation outputs, on a very high number of very short poles. The companies supplying 5G might first put 4G on the poles, calling it 5GE (evolution) or 4LTE to try to alleviate 5G fears and get its equipment into the field early, and then convert over to true 5G short wavelengths at a later date. Why is 5G being put in when fiber-optic cabling will be required to serve every one of those new antenna installed? Why is 5G being installed when fiber optics are safer health-wise, have more capacity, are secure and far faster?

At a U.S. Senate Commerce Hearing on February 7, 2019, Senator Richard Blumenthal of Connecticut raised serious concerns on 5G Wireless Technology's potential health risks. The Senator criticized both the FCC & FDA for inadequate answers on outstanding public health questions. At the meeting, representatives from all the major wireless carriers conceded they are unaware of any independent scientific studies on the safety of 5G technologies. www.blumenthal.senate.gov/newsroom/press/release/at-senate-commerce-hearing-blumenthal-raises-concerns-on-5g-wireless-technologys-potential-health-risks.

We need every citizen to be aware of the many health dangers of 5G. If we are complacent, we will be an enabler in the poisoning

by industry of our humanity. You will not have a choice to the dangerous health implications. The industry is holding hands with the people we voted into office. The communications industry is sending 20,000 satellites, 10 per rocket, with focused beams emitting 5G radiation into space to float above us 24/7.
www.cellphonetaskforce.org/planetary-emergency

To see if your transient symptoms might be related to an overhead Google Loon balloon, see online site
www.flightradar24.com/34.43,-112.19/9.

There is new information everyday on the health ramifications of 5G. I you would like more information:
www.mdsafetech.org/news.
www.whatis5g.info/
www.ehtrust.org/wp-content/uploads/Scientist-5G-appeal-2017.pdf
www.electricsense.com/12399/5g-radiation-dangers

    There is no longer a place to go without microwave radiation. We, in our complacency, are creating a nightmarish society of disillusioned non-social beings. I personally think the government likes it like that. We are totally radiated with towers, drones, satellites, and balloons. Our information is being mined and we will not have the freedom or the ability to be on our own, as the surveillance of our every move is now tracked or traced.
    When did we lose the ability to make decisions about the health and safety of ourselves and our environment? Scary times, but we are strong and we aren't alone; there are many that believe as we do. I think that the greatest gift I can give to myself, family, and grand babies is a protest against the injustices brought on by those willing to bow to industry. I will write letters, send emails, make posters, and phone my elected officials. We need to stand up to this travesty, this crime, against

humanity. Find your unique way, and join me, please. When enough of us stand together, our voices will be heard.

Note: Due to the dismantling of Net Neutrality (Open Internet) by the FCC, many of the websites I list may not be available. Even in the short writing of this chapter, several sites have gone "404, page not found". Our Open Internet of things is being monitored, screened, and information hidden. We are losing "Freedom of Information." If a link you click on appears "404," copy the link and put it directly into search and it usually appears.

Just because we can do all things wireless, doesn't mean we should.

White Zones

Due to outside sources of wireless radiation, some EHS or Microwave Sickness sufferers are no longer able to live in their homes. They look for what all others take for granted: a good night's sleep and pain free living. Many EMF Refugees have had to resort to living in their vehicles in secluded areas or camping in wilderness areas. They have no other recourse than to leave behind all they have known for health reasons. Many EHS sufferers have had to desert modern living in search of a viable solution for healthy living. Many have no other choice but to leave a job that was causing illness, and as a result, have lost their home. Safe living for those sensitive to man-made environmental hazards is a most important issue that needs to be addressed by lawmakers.

A White Zone, also known as an "EMF Quiet Zone", is an area free of EMF set aside for those suffering from EHS. At this time, white zones are very primitive properties usually without conveniences such as electricity or toilets. These seem to be just open land for setting up housekeeping and safe from EMF sources. Europe is ahead of the United States in awareness of the hazards of EMF. France used to have a White Zone that was open to EHS sufferers to bring their own small RV trailer for limited time camping. This was offered so they might recover from a poisoning, recoup some health, and build up their immune system. So many have become sensitive and fled to this area, they are no longer accepting new lodgers. Italy used to have a White Zone, but a company put up a cell tower nearby, so it is now defunct. In Australia there is a "radio quiet zone" supporting a large radio telescope. Supposedly there are two sites being developed in British Columbia, and one White Zone in Spain under development. As of this writing, the United States has one in Snowflake Arizona. There are a couple other sites that are hoping to set up as a "White Zone, two being developed in Arizona, one in southeastern Utah, one in Grass Valley,

California, and one in Rockvale, Colorado. I am sure that demand for these safe areas will skyrocket in conjunction with the climbing rate of EHS sufferers.

Greenbank, West Virginia, where the world's largest steerable radio telescope is located, restricts wireless transmissions by law. Because of this restriction, Greenbank is considered a White Zone or "radio free zone" by EMF Refugees. It is not known just how long this radio telescope will remain in operation, as it relies on government funding. There is a growing demand from some Greenbank citizens for wireless conveniences, and Big Wireless is chomping at the bit to EMF Up this whole area. For now, Greenbank has "radio policemen" who patrol with a radiation meter on the lookout for EMF usurpers.

It would be wonderful if those with EHS joined together and created a safe haven. Sadly, I believe it would be quite difficult to find a plot of land without EMF. There must be little canyons or areas overlooked by the telecom industry that might be safe, but I personally don't know of any. I have approached real estate agents that deal with rural property and have asked them to keep an eye out for any properties that might get poor cell reception, thinking this might be a starting place to look and test with the meter. I don't know whether they can't find any property as described or they think I am nuts, as I never hear back.

I know I've mentioned that one of the worst places to find yourself, is when you are ill and have to go to the hospital or to the doctor's office. I delay seeing a physician because a doctor's office is one of the places with the highest levels of radiation we have read. I believe that every clinic, physician's office, emergency room and hospital **should be mandated** to have rooms safe White Zone rooms for the EHS and MCS. I have contacted the UCSF hospital and spoken with several heads of departments, always being handed off to a different person when they hear that I would like them to consider a white zone room where those with MCS and EHS may be seen in relative ease. UCSF stated they are unaware of an issue and declined. I found out that they might consider a home visit. It would be a good idea to approach this subject with your personal physician, as a home visit may be a preferred option to maintain health care.

Italian courts voted to initiate a public awareness campaign beginning July of 2019, regarding hazards of EMF and its sources. The U.S. will not make this stand, but together as EHS survivors, maybe we can spread awareness. We deserve the right to be able to avoid these exposures. We deserve a safe place to live. Isn't that a part of "life, liberty and the pursuit of happiness"?

To read the plights of EHS Refugees, or to add your story, visit www.emfanalysis.com/emf-refugee
For information on International White Zones, visit www.emf-experts.com/emf-quiet-zones.html

Take-Aways

After reading this book, my hope would be that you are more aware of microwave radiation's harmful effects and be more accepting of those with EHS. As a society, we need to insist that our physicians are trained in adverse environmental impacts on health. We need to start finding ways to set aside safe places for our wireless sensitized population.

Our society has a new bogey man and we are the makers, the enablers. By not investigating what we were bringing into our home, what we were saying "yes" to, we unexpectedly granted permission to the EMF that now permeate our whole world's culture. We have poisoned our environment. Radiation is at a point where a great percentage of our society will be unable to live safely in most places on earth. This is no exaggeration. We need to insist on independent scientific medical studies on the detrimental health effects of EMF. We must make White Zones for safe living. If we are to continue as a people, we must start to be aware of, limit, and greatly reduce man made pulsed microwave radiation.

1. Avoid EMF wherever possible. Use tech devices prudently. Use a cord.
2. Get a meter and learn to use it.
3. Protect yourself. Protect your home, auto, work place.
4. Eat and drink organic, exercise, take necessary supplements.
5. Learn all you can about EMFs and EHS, and learn to be situationally aware.
6. Document symptoms. Document EMF readings.
7. Teach your physicians. Teach your lawyers. Teach your children's teachers.
8. Talk. Share. Help others become aware of the dangers. Who can you help?
9. Know you are not alone. You are a survivor.

"There is no more neutrality in the world. You either have to be part of the solution, or you're going to be part of the problem."
Eldridge Cleaver, (1935-1998)
American writer and political activist.

Thank you.

Conclusion

To those with EHS, please know that though you may feel a victim, you are in a large club of Survivors. You are not alone. If you are a Shepherd of someone with EHS, I hope that in some small way I was able to help. To those who only see me in metalized veils, I hope I have answered any questions you might have, and please say hello when we meet. For those readers who were just curious, I hope we've helped you become a little more aware of EMFs so you may take steps to protect yourself and your loved ones.

Only with everyone's awareness, acknowledgement, and willingness to learn of the dangers and act accordingly, will we be able to clean up the environment we have poisoned. There is nowhere we can hide from the fact that the industry has us captured, and we will pay with our health and that of our children, pets, and our natural surroundings, unless we, together, make fast and drastic changes. Start with protecting yourself and your home, and talk to your partners, your children, your neighbors, and your doctor. Write to your elected officials. Talk to your child's teachers. Share the knowledge.

I would like to thank those in our small community for all their support of my affliction; by them turning their phones off, or refusing smart meters, they have allowed me to be present and a part of their lives. They have allowed me to live my life a little fuller in knowing them.

To my readers, Thank you for allowing me to share my experience. This book, and the possibility that it might help someone, is the only way I could feel that this life's event had any reason to take place.

Epilogue

I have a reoccurring nightmare…

I am walking down a narrow cement hallway, the harsh cement slams up against my shoes. The grey cold hallway is lined with large picture windows, as if I am in a giant store mall. In these windows are colorful scenes where I see people, some whom I know, enjoying each other's company over coffee, shopping with friends, or looking at books. I attempt to enter these stores and find that the doors are on the ground and no bigger than a coffee can. I watch as other people come by and magically they are able to enter the store through this tiny opening. I am not able to morph through this coffee-can opening. I try to fit my foot in the opening, I try to enter, but for some reason, denied.

Every night this dream plays out; not always the same store, or the same people, but if there were an instance where I wanted to enter, shop, or accompany someone in a social event, I am stymied by a coffee-can entrance. I am left in a gray cement hallway with windows, and I am always looking in.

Anne Mills

More Info

Many with EHS, due to their particular sensitivities, are unable to work on a computer. I have been fortunate in that my computer is on a cable, and the mouse, keyboard, all computer equipment, is wired. I have given most of the resources in online sources, which makes it difficult for those who do not have a computer at their disposal, and so I apologize. For those who are unable to use or do not have a computer, I have listed a few books on EHS.

For those who are able to use a computer, all it takes is a good search. There are many sites showing "dangers of electromagnetic fields". You are lucky. When I first became ill in 2006, and for several years after, there wasn't much information on EHS. I wish there had been all this information, as I would not have felt so alone. There are now many video's on YouTube and sites online. There are an increasing number of books written by not only those that suffer from EHS, but written by scientists and doctors intent on bringing awareness of the dangers of EMF to the public.

Books: There are quite a few books on EHS. I have not read all books listed.

The Invisible Rainbow: A History of Electricity and Life, by Arthur Firstenberg (ACH Press, 2017) This book is very easy to read, full of interesting history relating to energy, great insights into how man opened Pandora's box of energy induced health ramifications. Wonderfully researched book. (Great book - A must read!)

Overpowered, by Martin Blank

Wireless Radiation Rescue, by Kerry Crofton, PhD. (Wonderful book!)

Non-Tinfoil-Guide-EMFs-StupidTechnology by Nicholas Pineault

Exposed: The Electronic Sickening of America by Bill Cadwallader

Disconnect: The Truth About Cell Phone Radiation, What the Industry Has Done to Hide It, and How to Protect Your Family by Devra Davis

Doubt is Their Product: How Industry Scientists Manufacture Uncertainty and Threaten Your Health by David Michaels

Cellphones and Brain Tumors: 15 Reasons for Concern by Lloyd Morgan
Science, Spin and the Truth Behind Interphone, by Lloyd Morgan

YouTube Video's and Movies

Generation Zapped This movie has won many awards.

There are many wonderful short you tube videos on 'electrosensitivity' or EHS,:
You Tube: Toril Jelter, Pediatrician (Health effects of non ionizing radiation on children)

This is not a tree, by B. Theldea shows one person's discovery of EMF and their efforts at protecting themselves.

"Searching for a Golden Cage," is a short film depicting several EHS sufferers and their search for a place to live without EMF radiation.

Favorite WebSites to name a few:
www.emfsafetynetwork.org
www.ehtrust.org
www.wiredchild.org
www.MagdaHavas.com
www.SaferEMR.com
www.CitizensForSafeTechnology.org
www.mdsafetech.org
www.Smartmeterharm.org
www.Emfanalysis.com
www.scientists4wiredtech.com
www.electrosensitivity.co (not com)
www.bioinitiative.org
https://www.electricsense.com/2431/smart-meter-shielding-tips
www.cellphonetaskforce.org
www.ehs-mcs.org (EHS and MCS Research and Treatment European Group)
www.researchgate.net/profile/Joel_Moskowitz
www.electromagnetichealth.org/
www.ehsidaho.com
www.wearetheevidence.org   We are the Evidence

Studies. Many studies can be found at the above sites, or :

Reliable disease biomarkers characterizing and identifying electrohypersensitivity and multiple chemical sensitivity as two etiopathogenic aspects of a unique pathological disorder.
https://www.ncbi.nlm.nih.gov/pubmed/26613326

A resource to educate your physician is EUROPAEM EMF Guideline 2016 for the prevention, diagnosis and treatment of

EMF-related health problems and illnesses
https://www.degruyter.com/view/j/reveh.2016.31.issue-3/reveh-2016-0011/reveh-2016-0011.xml (Look under the tab "Electromagnetic Sensitivity" for other resources)
>Groups affiliated with the report include Powerwatch, EM Radiation Research Trust in the UK, EMR Policy Institute, ElectromagneticHealth.org, and The Peoples Initiative Foundation in the US.

Information on EMF and our Environment
Our pets living depends on us, and in our lifestyle choices we are unthinkingly subjecting them to radiation. They are as susceptible to EMF as ourselves and our children. Our lifestyles and choices affect the nature that our environment supports, having a huge ripple effect. The following sites offer perspectives we might want to consider in our choices.
https://www.mainecoalitiontostopsmartmeters.org/wp-content/uploads/2015/08/India-final_mobile_towers_wildlife-report.pdf

https://mdsafetech.org/environmental-and-wildlife-effects/

Notes:

Notes:

Notes: